a LANGE medical book

CURRENT
Practice Guidelines
In Primary Care
2008

Ralph Gonzales, MD, MSPH

Professor of Medicine
Division of General Internal Medicine
University of California, San Francisco
San Francisco, California

Jean S. Kutner, MD, MSPH

Associate Professor of Medicine and Division Head
Division of General Internal Medicine
University of Colorado at Denver, and Health Sciences Center
Denver, Colorado

D1402264

 Medical

New York   Chicago   San Francisco   Lisbon   London
Madrid   Mexico City   Milan   New Delhi   San Juan   Seoul
Singapore   Sydney   Toronto

CURRENT Practice Guidelines in Primary Care, 2008

1 2 3 4 5 6 7 8 9 0 DOC/DOC 0 9 8 7

ISBN 978-007-149634-6
MHID 0-07-1496343
ISSN 1528-1612

Notice

This book was set in Times New Roman by Silverchair Science + Communications, Inc. The editor was Ruth Weinberg.
The production supervisor was Thomas Kowalczyk.
Project management was provided by Silverchair Science + Communications, Inc. RR Donnelley was printer and binder.

This book is printed on acid-free paper.

Contents

1. DISEASE SCREENING

√ denotes major 2008 updates.
+ denotes new topic for 2008.

√ denotes major 2008 updates.
+ denotes new topic for 2008.

2. DISEASE PREVENTION

3. DISEASE MANAGEMENT

√ denotes major 2008 updates.
+ denotes new topic for 2008.

√ denotes major 2008 updates.
+ denotes new topic for 2008.

4. APPENDICES

√ denotes major 2008 updates.
+ denotes new topic for 2008.

Preface

Current Practice Guidelines in Primary Care, 2008 is intended for primary care clinicians, including not only residents and practicing physicians in the specialties of family medicine, internal medicine, pediatrics, and obstetrics and gynecology, but also medical and nursing students during their ambulatory care rotations, registered nurses, nurse practitioners, and physician assistants. Its purpose is to make screening, prevention, and management recommendations readily accessible and available for clinical decision making. The recommendations included are issued by governmental agencies, expert panels, medical specialty organizations, and other professional and scientific organizations.

Current Practice Guidelines in Primary Care, 2008 is essential for the busy clinician. New recommendations are continually being published by various organizations that express different positions on the same topics, and current guidelines require revision as new evidence from clinical and outcomes research emerges. Indeed, we update or completely revise approximately 40% of *Current Practice Guidelines in Primary Care* each year. The intent of this guide is both to help clinicians select the most appropriate clinical services and interventions for a given situation and to provide clinicians with quick access to the latest information.

Current Practice Guidelines in Primary Care, 2008 has been updated using PubMed searches limited to articles published in English between 7/24/06 and 7/20/07, as well as via the websites of and contact with the major professional societies, the Agency for Healthcare Research and Quality "Guidelines Clearinghouse," and the U.S. Preventive Services Task Force. This updating strategy led to substantial modification of many guidelines (look for "√" in the Contents). New material includes new topics on developmental dysplasia of the hip, asymptomatic gonorrhea infection, asymptomatic genital herpes simplex, and speech and language delay.

New screening and prevention guidelines have been added for the following topics:

- Abdominal aortic aneurysm
- Alcohol abuse and dependence
- Breast, cervical, colorectal, liver, and prostate cancer
- Carotid artery stenosis
- Chlamydial infection
- Cholesterol screening in children and adolescents
- Coronary artery disease screening and primary prevention
- Endocarditis
- Hemochromatosis
- Hepatitis B and C infection
- HIV
- Hypertension screening and primary prevention
- Lead poisoning
- Obesity in children and adolescents
- Osteoporotic hip fracture prevention
- Visual impairment in children

Disease Management Guidelines with new or major updates include:
- Atrial fibrillation
- Asthma
- Cholesterol and lipid management in children
- Metabolic syndrome
- Stable COPD management
- Diabetes management
- Hypertension in children and adolescents
- Obesity management
- Pap smear abnormalities
- Perioperative cardiovascular evaluation
- Community-acquired pneumonia
- Childhood, adolescent, and adult immunizations

European guidelines have been added for the following topics:
- Breast, cervical, and colorectal cancer screening
- Coronary artery disease screening
- Depression screening
- Diabetes screening
- Hepatitis B and C screening
- Hypertension screening
- Obesity screening
- Endocarditis prevention
- Osteoporotic hip fracture prevention
- Stable COPD management
- Pap smear abnormalities

We are grateful to Karen Mellis for her assistance in contacting and obtaining information from professional societies and updating internet addresses, as well as the following professional societies for providing updates/feedback on their content: AAFP, AAHPM, AAN, AAP, ACC, ACCP, ACP, ACR, AGS, AHA, ASGE, CDC, ICSI, JCIH, CTF, NAPNAP, NICE, ACIP, NIAAA, USPSTF, and USSG.

Ralph Gonzales, MD, MSPH
Professor of Medicine
University of California, San Francisco
San Francisco, California

Jean S. Kutner, MD, MSPH
Associate Professor of Medicine and Division Head
University of Colorado at Denver, and Health Sciences Center
Denver, Colorado

December 2007

1
Disease Screening

ABDOMINAL AORTIC ANEURYSM						
Disease Screening	Organization	Date	Population	Recommendations	Comments	Source
Abdominal Aortic Aneurysm	USPSTF	2005	Men aged 65–75 years who have ever smoked	One-time screening for AAA by ultrasonography. No recommendation for or against screening for AAA in men aged 65–75 who have never smoked.	1. Surgical repair of AAA ≥ 5.5 cm reduces AAA-specific mortality in men aged 65–75 years who have ever smoked. 2. Unclear benefit-harm ratio in men aged 65–75 who have never smoked. 3. Cochrane review (2007): Significant decrease in AAA-specific mortality in men (OR, 0.60, 95% CI 0.47–0.99) but not for women. (Cochrane Database of Syst Rev 2007;2:CD002945; http://www.thecochranelibrary.com)	http://www.ahrq.gov/clinic/uspstf/uspsaneu.htm
	USPSTF	2005	Women	Routine screening is not recommended.	4. Early mortality benefit of screening (men aged 65–74 years) maintained at 7-year follow-up. Cost-effectiveness of screening improves over time. (Ann Intern Med 2007;146:699)	
	CSVS	2007	Men aged 65–75 years who are candidates for surgery	Recommend population-based screening using ultrasonography.	5. Among patients with AAA ≥ 5.5 cm considered medically fit for open surgery, endovascular repair has greater short- and long-term costs with no improvement in overall survival or quality of life beyond 1 year. (Intl J of Technol Assess 2007;23:205–215)	J Vasc Surg 2007;45:1268–1276

ALCOHOL ABUSE & DEPENDENCE

Disease Screening	Organization	Date	Population	Recommendations	Comments	Source
Alcohol Abuse & Dependence	USPSTF	2004	Adolescents	Evidence is insufficient to recommend for or against screening and behavioral counseling interventions to prevent or reduce alcohol misuse by adolescents in primary care settings.	1. Parents should routinely receive instructions on monitoring their adolescent's social and recreational activities for use of alcohol.[a] 2. The finding of alcohol use or abuse should provoke an assessment of other conditions that co-vary with alcohol abuse, such as cigarette smoking, sexual activity, and mood disorders. 3. Guidelines on treatment of alcohol abuse in adolescence have been published. (*J Am Acad Child Adolesc Psychiatry* 1998;37:122)	http://www.ahrq.gov/clinic/uspstf/uspsdrin.htm
	BrightFutures	2002	Adolescents	Ask all adolescents annually about their use of alcohol.		http://www.brightfutures.org

Disease Screening	Organization	Date	Population	Recommendations	Comments	Source
ALCOHOL ABUSE & DEPENDENCE						
Alcohol Abuse & Dependence (continued)	NIAAA	2002	College students	Screen all students on National Alcohol Screening Day.[b]	1. 1,400 college students between the ages of 18 and 24 die each year from alcohol-related injuries. (J Studies Alcohol 2002;63:136) 2. Targeting only those with identified problems misses students who drink heavily or misuse alcohol occasionally. Nondependent, high-risk drinkers account for majority of alcohol-related deaths and damage. 3. In 2001, 18% of U.S. college students had clinically significant alcohol-related problems in the past year. [Arch Gen Psychiatry 2005 Mar;62(3):321]	http://www.collegedrinking prevention.gov
	NIAAA	2007	Adults	Screen all adults for heavy drinking (see Appendix). Assess heavy drinkers for alcohol use disorders.[c] Advise and assist with a brief intervention (see Management). Continue support at follow-up visits.	1. A free guide, including a pocket version and patient education handouts, of "Helping patients who drink too much: a clinician's guide" is available at http://www.niaaa.nih.gov, or by calling 301-443-3860. 2. The COMBINE study reported better 16-week abstinence rates with medical management using naltrexone, but not acamprosate. Combined behavioral intervention (CBI) plus placebo medical management was also more effective than CBI alone. There was no difference between any groups in abstinence rates at 1-year follow-up. (JAMA 2006;295:2003)	http://www.niaaa.nih.gov

ALCOHOL ABUSE & DEPENDENCE

Disease Screening	Organization	Date	Population	Recommendations	Comments	Source
Alcohol Abuse & Dependence (continued)	AAFP USPSTF	2007 2004	Adults	Screen all adults, including pregnant women, using relevant history or a standardized screening instrument. Implement brief behavioral counseling interventions to reduce alcohol misuse.[c]	1. A systematic review concluded that the Alcohol Use Disorders Identification Test (AUDIT) was most useful for identifying subjects with at-risk, hazardous, or harmful drinking (sensitivity, 51%–79%; specificity, 78%–96%) while the CAGE questions proved superior for detecting alcohol abuse and dependence (sensitivity, 43%–94%; specificity, 70%–97%). (Arch Intern Med 2000;160:1977)[d] 2. The USPSTF found two poor-to-fair quality studies indicating that screening coupled with brief physician advice is cost-effective. (Ann Intern Med 2004;140:558–569)	Ann Intern Med 2004;140:557 http://www.ahrq.gov/clinic/uspstf/uspdrin.htm http://www.aafp.org/online/en/home/clinical/exam.html
	AGS	2003	Adults aged ≥ 65 years	Ask about use of alcohol at least annually.	3. Light to moderate alcohol consumption has been associated with some health benefits in middle-aged or older adults, including reduced risk for coronary artery disease.	http://www.americangeriatrics.org/products/positionpapers/alcohol.shtml

[a]The importance of family attitudes toward alcohol is also acknowledged, and it is recommended that clinicians urge parents to use alcohol safely and in moderation, to restrict children from family alcohol supplies, and to recognize the influence their own drinking patterns can have on their children and parenting.
[b]National Alcohol Screening Day is sponsored by the National Institute on Alcohol Abuse and Alcoholism and other organizations. (http://mentalhealthscreening.org/events/nasd/)
[c]Hazardous drinking is defined as more than 7 drinks per week for women and more than 14 drinks per week for men. Harmful drinking describes people with physical, social, or psychological harm from drinking who do not meet criteria for dependence. (Arch Intern Med 1999;159)
[d]See Appendix I: Screening Instruments, Alcohol Abuse for CAGE and AUDIT instruments.

Disease Screening	Organization	Date	Population	Recommendations	Comments	Source
Anemia	AAFP	2006	Infants aged 6–12 months	Perform selective, single hemoglobin or hematocrit screening for high-risk infants.[a]	1. Reticulocyte hemoglobin content is a more sensitive marker than serum hemoglobin level for iron deficiency.	http://www.aafp.org/online/en/home/clinical/exam.html
	USPSTF	2006	Infants aged 6–12 months	Evidence is insufficient to recommend for or against routine screening.	1. Recommends routine iron supplementation in high-risk children aged 6–12 months.	
	USPSTF	2006	Pregnant women	Screen all women with hemoglobin or hematocrit at first prenatal visit.	1. Insufficient evidence to recommend for or against routine use of iron supplements for non-anemic pregnant women. (USPSTF) 2. When acute stress or inflammatory disorders are not present, a serum ferritin level is the most accurate test for evaluating iron deficiency anemia. Among women of childbearing age, a cut-off of 15 mg/dL has sensitivity of 75%, specificity of 98%. (Br J Haematol 1993;85:787)	http://www.ahrq.gov/clinic/cpsix.htm

[a]Includes infants living in poverty, blacks, Native Americans and Alaska Natives, immigrants from developing countries, preterm and low birthweight infants, and infants whose principal dietary intake is unfortified cow's milk.

ATTENTION-DEFICIT/HYPERACTIVITY DISORDER

Disease Screening	Organization	Date	Population	Recommendations	Comments	Source
Attention-Deficit/ Hyperactivity Disorder (ADHD)	AAFP AAP	2000	Children aged 6–12 years with inattention, hyperactivity, impulsivity, academic under-achievement, or behavioral problems	Initiate an evaluation for ADHD. Diagnosis requires the child meet DSM IV criteria,[a] and direct supporting evidence from parents or caregivers and classroom teacher. Evaluation of child with ADHD should include assessment for coexisting disorders.	1. The sharp rise in stimulant prescriptions between 1987 and 1996 plateaued between 1996 and 2002. In 2002, 4.8% of 6–12-year-olds received stimulant therapy, compared with 3.2% of 13–19-year-olds. (Am J Psychiatr 2006;163:579) 2. An estimated 4.4% of the U.S. adult population meets criteria for ADHD; large majority is undiagnosed and untreated. (Am J Psychiatr 2006;163: 716) 3. The FDA recently approved a "black box" warning regarding the potential for cardiovascular side effects of ADHD stimulant drugs. (NEJM 2006;354:1445)	Pediatrics 2000;105:1158

[a]DSM-IV Criteria for ADHD: I: Either A or B. A: *Six or more of the following symptoms of inattention have been present for at least 6 months to a point that is disruptive and inappropriate for developmental level. Inattention:* (1) Often does not give close attention to details or makes careless mistakes in schoolwork, work, or other activities. (2) Often has trouble keeping attention on tasks or play activities. (3) Often does not seem to listen when spoken to directly. (4) Often does not follow instructions and fails to finish schoolwork, chores, or duties in the workplace (not due to oppositional behavior or failure to understand instructions). (5) Often has trouble organizing activities. (6) Often avoids, dislikes, or doesn't want to do things that take a lot of mental effort for a long period of time (such as schoolwork or homework). (7) Often loses things needed for tasks and activities (eg, toys, school assignments, pencils, books, or tools). (8) Is often easily distracted. (9) Is often forgetful in daily activities. B: *Six or more of the following symptoms of hyperactivity-impulsivity have been present for at least 6 months to an extent that is disruptive and inappropriate for developmental level. Hyperactivity:* (1) Often fidgets with hands or feet or squirms in seat. (2) Often gets up from seat when remaining in seat is expected. (3) Often runs about or climbs when and where it is not appropriate (adolescents or adults may feel very restless). (4) Often has trouble playing or enjoying leisure activities quietly. (5) Is often "on the go" or often acts as if "driven by a motor." (6) Often talks excessively. *Impulsivity:* (1) Often blurts out answers before questions have been finished. (2) Often has trouble waiting one's turn. (3) Often interrupts or intrudes on others (eg, butts into conversations or games). II: Some symptoms that cause impairment were present before age 7 years. III: There must be clear evidence of significant impairment in social, school, or work functioning. V: The symptoms do not happen only during the course of a Pervasive Developmental Disorder, Schizophrenia, or other Psychotic Disorder. The symptoms are not better accounted for by another mental disorder (eg, Mood Disorder, Anxiety Disorder, Dissociative Disorder, or a Personality Disorder).

CANCER, BLADDER

Disease Screening	Organization	Date	Population	Recommendations	Comments	Source
Cancer, Bladder	AAFP USPSTF	2007 2004	Asymptomatic persons	Recommends against routine screening for bladder cancer in adults.	1. *Benefits:* There is inadequate evidence to determine whether screening for bladder cancer would have any impact on mortality. *Harms:* Based on fair evidence, screening for bladder cancer would result in unnecessary diagnostic procedures with attendant morbidity. (NCI, 2007) 2. A high index of suspicion should be maintained in anyone with a history of smoking or exposure to another risk factor.[a] 3. Decision analysis of total cost of screening for bladder cancer using NMP22: (1) Screening all men, regardless of degree of risk, yields cost per cancer detected of $783,913, $269,028, and $139,305 for ages 50–59, 60–69, and 70–79 years, respectively. (2) Screening only high-risk yields cost per cancer detected of $3,310. [Urol Oncol 2006;24(4):338]	http://www.aafp.org/online/en/home/clinical/exam.html http://www.ahrq.gov/clinic/uspstf/uspsblad.htm http://www.cancer.gov/cancer_information/testing

[a]Individuals who smoke are four to seven times more likely to develop bladder cancer than individuals who have never smoked. Additional environmental risk factors: exposure to aminobiphenyls; aromatic amines; azodyes; combustion gases and soot from coal; chlorination byproducts in heated water; aldehydes used in chemical dyes and in the rubber and textile industries; organic chemicals used in dry cleaning, paper manufacturing, rope and twine making, and apparel manufacturing; contaminated Chinese herbs; arsenic in well water. Additional risk factors: prolonged exposure to urinary *Schistosoma haematobium* bladder infections, cyclophosphamide, or pelvic radiation therapy for other malignancies.

Disease Screening	Organization	Date	Population	Recommendations[a,b]	Comments	Source
CANCER, BREAST						
Cancer, Breast	ACS	2007	Women aged 20–39 years	Inform women of risks and benefits of breast self-exam (BSE). Clinician breast exam (CBE).	1. *Benefits of mammography screening:* Based on fair evidence, screening mammography in women aged 40–70 years decreases breast cancer mortality. *Harms:* Based on solid evidence, screening mammography may lead to harms in Table A. (See page 14.) (NCI, 2007)	http://www.cancer.org
	ACP	2007	Women aged 40–49 years	Perform individualized assessment of breast cancer risk every 1–2 years; base screening decision on benefits and harms of screening (see Comment 1) as well as on a woman's preferences and cancer risk profile.	2. Breast self-examination does not improve breast cancer mortality (Br J Cancer 2003;88:1047) and increases the rate of false-positive biopsies. (J Natl Cancer Inst 2002;94:1445) 3. 25% of breast cancers diagnosed before age 40 years are attributable to *BRCA1* mutations. 4. Breast cancer-specific mortality is reduced by 20%–35% by mammography screening in women aged 50–69 years. (NEJM 2003;348:1672)	Ann Intern Med 2007;146:511
	UK-NHS	2006	Women aged 40–49 years	Based on current evidence, routine screening is not recommended.	5. Annual screening of young (age 35–49 years old) high-risk women with MRI and mammography is superior to either alone. (Lancet 2005;365:1769) 6. Computer-aided detection in screening mammography appears to reduce overall accuracy (by increasing false-positive rate). (NEJM 2007;356:1399)	http://www.cancerscreening.nhs.uk

CANCER, BREAST

Disease Screening	Organization	Date	Population	Recommendations[a,b]	Comments	Source
Cancer, Breast (continued)	WHO	2007	Women aged ≥ 40 years	Encourage early diagnosis of breast cancer, especially for women aged 40–69 years. (1) Offer clinical breast exams to those concerned about their breasts, and for promoting awareness in the community. (2) If mammography is available, the top priority is to use it for diagnosis, especially for women who have detected an abnormality by self-examination. (3) Mammography should not be introduced for screening unless the resources are available to ensure effective and reliable sreening of at least 70% of the target age group, that is, women over the age of 50 years.		http://www.who.int/cancer/detection/breastcancer/en/index.html

CANCER, BREAST					
Disease Screening	Organization	Date	Population	Recommendations[a,b]	Comments	Source
Cancer, Breast (continued)	AAFP USPSTF	2007 2002	Women aged ≥ 40 years	Mammography, with or without CBE, every 1–2 years after counseling about potential risks and benefits.	Evidence is insufficient to recommend for or against routine CBE alone, or teaching or performing routine BSE.	http://www.aafp.org/online/en/home/clinical/exam.html http://www.ahrq.gov/clinic/uspstf/uspsbrca.htm
	ACS	2007	Women aged ≥ 40 years	Mammography and CBE yearly; if > 20% lifetime risk of breast cancer, annual mammogram + MRI.		http://www.cancer.org
	UK-NHS	2006	Women aged 50–70 years Women aged > 70 years	Program-initiated mammography screening of all women every 3 years. Patient-initiated screening covered by NHS.	Annual vs. 3-year screening interval showed no significant difference in predicted breast cancer mortality, although relative risk reduction among annually screened women had point estimates of –5% to –11%. (Eur J Cancer 2002;38:1458)	http://www.cancerscreening.nhs.uk

CANCER, BREAST						
Disease Screening	**Organization**	**Date**	**Population**	**Recommendations**[a,b]	**Comments**	**Source**
Cancer, Breast (continued)	AGS	2005	Women aged 70–85 years	If estimated life expectancy ≥ 5 years, then offer screening mammography ± CBE every 1–2 years.		http://www.americangeriatrics.org/products/positionpapers/breast_cancer_position_statement.pdf
	AAFP USPSTF	2007 2005	Women with family history associated with increased risk for deleterious mutations in *BRCA1* or *BRCA2* genes[c,d]	Refer for genetic counseling and evaluation for *BRCA* testing.	In one study, nearly half of *BRCA*-positive women developed malignant disease detected by mammography less than 1 year after a normal screening mammogram. (Cancer 2004; 100:2079)	http://www.aafp.org/online/en/home/clinical/exam.html http://www.ahrq.gov/clinic/uspstf/uspstfbrgen.htm

CANCER, BREAST

Disease Screening	Organization	Date	Population	Recommendations[a,b]	Comments	Source
Cancer, Breast (continued)	COG	2006	Chest radiation (≥ 20 Gy to mantle, mini-mantle, medi-astinal, chest, axilla)	Yearly mammogram beginning 8 years after radiation, or at age 25, whichever occurs last.		http://www.survivorshipguidelines.org

[a]Debate about the value of screening mammograms was triggered by a Cochrane review published on October 20, 2001. (Lancet 2001;358:1340–1342) This review cited a number of methodologic and analytic flaws in the large long-term mammography trials. The USPSTF and NCI concluded that the flaws were problematic but unlikely to negate the consistent and significant mortality reductions observed in the trials.

[b]Summary of current evidence: JAMA 2005;293:1245.

[c](1) Women not of Ashkenazi Jewish heritage:

- Two first-degree relatives with breast cancer, 1 of whom received the diagnosis at age ≤ 50 years
- A combination of ≥ 3 first- or second-degree relatives with breast cancer
- A combination of both breast and ovarian cancer among first- and second-degree relatives
- A first-degree relative with bilateral breast cancer
- A combination of ≥ 2 first- or second-degree relatives with ovarian cancer
- A first- or second-degree relative with both breast and ovarian cancer
- A history of breast cancer in a male relative

(2) Women of Ashkenazi Jewish heritage: Any first-degree relative (or 2 second-degree relatives on the same side of the family) with breast or ovarian cancer

[d]USPSTF recommends against routine referral for genetic couseling or routine *BRCA* testing of women without a family history associated with increase risk for deleterious mutations in *BRCA1* or *BRCA2* genes.

CANCER, BREAST				
TABLE A: HARMS OF SCREENING MAMMOGRAPHY				
Harm	**Internal Validity**	**Consistency**	**Magnitude of Effects**	**External Validity**
Treatment of insignificant cancers (overdiagnosis, true positives) can result in breast deformity, lymph-edema, thromboembolic events, new cancers, or chemotherapy-induced toxicities.	Good	Good	Approximately 33% of breast cancers detected by screening mammograms represent overdiagnosis. (BMJ 2004;328:921–924)	Good
Additional testing (false-positives)	Good	Good	Estimated to occur in 50% of women screened annually for 10 years, 25% of whom will have biopsies. (NEJM 1998;338:1089–1096)	Good
False sense of security, delay in cancer diagnosis (false-negatives)	Good	Good	6% to 46% of women with invasive cancer will have negative mammograms, especially if young, with dense breasts (Radiology 1998;209:511–518, JAMA 1996;276:39–43), or with mucinous, lobular, or fast-growing cancers. (J Natl Cancer Inst 1991;91:2020–2028)	Good
Radiation-induced mutation can cause breast cancer, especially if exposed before age 30 years. Latency is more than 10 years, and the increased risk persists lifelong.	Good	Good	Between 9.9 and 32 breast cancers per 10,000 women exposed to a cumulative dose of 1 Sv. Risk is higher for younger women.	Good
Source: NCI, 2007.				

					CANCER, CERVICAL	

Disease Screening	Organization	Date	Population	Recommendations	Comments	Source
Cancer, Cervical	ACS	2007	Women within 3 years after first sexual intercourse or by age 21, whichever comes first[a]	Annual Pap smear until age 30 (every 2 years if liquid-based Pap test). (ACS)[b] At age ≥ 30, if 3 consecutive normal Paps, may screen with Pap every 2–3 years; or screen every 3 years with Pap plus HPV DNA test. Continue to screen annually if risk factors present.[c]	1. Cervical cancer is causally related to infection with HPV. 2. Long-term use of oral contraceptives may increase risk of cervical cancer in women who are positive for cervical human papillomavirus DNA. (Lancet 2002;359:1085) 3. A vaccine against HPV-16 significantly reduces the risk of acquiring transient and persistent infection and cervical cancer. [NEJM 2002;347:1645; Obstet Gynecol 2006;107(1)4] 4. *Benefits:* Based on solid evidence, regular screening of appropriate women with the Pap test reduces mortality from cervical cancer. Screening is effective when started within 3 years after first vaginal intercourse. *Harms:* Based on solid evidence, regular screening with the Pap test leads to additional diagnostic procedures and treatment for low-grade squamous intraepithelial lesions (LSILs), with uncertain long-term consequences on fertility and pregnancy. Harms are greatest for younger women, who have a higher prevalence of LSILs. LSILs often regress without treatment. (NCI, 2007)	http://www.cancer.org http://www.survivorship guidelines.org
	AAFP USPSTF	2007 2003	Women who have ever had sex and have a cervix[a]	Strongly recommends Pap smear at least every 3 years.[d]		http://www.aafp.org/online/en/home/clinical/exam.html http://www.ahrq.gov/clinic/uspstf/uspscerv.htm

Disease Screening	Organization	Date	Population	Recommendations	Comments	Source
Cancer, Cervical (continued)					5. New Technologies for Cervical Cancer screening trial compared conventional cytology (Pap) vs. liquid-based cytology and testing for high-risk HPV types: (1) liquid-based and conventional cytology showed similar sensitivity for detecting CIN; (2) liquid-based cytology increased proportion classified as ASCUS, LSIL, and HSIL; (3) HPV testing for high-risk types was more sensitive than both conventional and liquid-based cytology; (4) HPV testing alone with triage of HPV-positive women by cytology may be reasonable approach. (J Natl Cancer Inst 2006;98:765; Lancet Oncol 2006;7:547) 6. NICE has recommended that liquid-based cytology should be used as the main way of preparing samples of cervical cells for screening. (http://guidance.nice.org.uk/TA69/?c=91496)	
	IARC UK-NHS	2005 2004	Women aged <25 years	Routine screening is not recommended.		http://screening.iarc.fr http://www.cancerscreening.nhs.uk

Disease Screening	Organization	Date	Population	Recommendations	Comments	Source
Cancer, Cervical (continued)	IARC UK-NHS	2005 2004	Women aged 25–49 years Women aged 50–64 years	Routinely screen every 3 years (IARC: if country has sufficient resources, otherwise every 5 years). Routinely screen every 5 years with conventional cytology.	UK-NHS contacts all eligible women who are registered with a primary care doctor.	http://screening.iarc.fr http://www.cancerscreening. nhs.uk
	IARC	2005	Women ≥ 65 years	Women who have always tested negative in an organized screening program should cease screening once they attain the age of 65 years.		http://screening.iarc.fr
	UK-NHS	2004	Women ≥ 65 years	Screen women who have not been screened since age 50 years, or who have had recent abnormal tests.	Stop screening after age 65 years if 3 consecutive normal tests.	http://www.cancerscreening. nhs.uk

CANCER, CERVICAL

Disease Screening	Organization	Date	Population	Recommendations	Comments	Source
Cancer, Cervical (continued)	USPSTF	2003	Women aged > 65 years	1. Recommends against routine screening if woman has had adequate recent screening and normal Pap smears and is not otherwise at high risk for cervical cancer.[c] 2. Discontinuation of cervical cancer screening in older women is appropriate, provided women have had adequate recent screening with normal Pap results. The optimal age to discontinue is not clear.	1. In one study, women 65 years of age and older were 21% less likely than younger women to ever have had a Pap test and 33% less likely to have had a Pap test recently. Physician recommendation is the strongest predictor of whether a woman receives a Pap test. (Ann Intern Med 2000;133:1021–1024) 2. Beyond age 70, there is little evidence for or against screening women who have been regularly screened in previous years. Individual circumstances, such as the patient's life expectancy, ability to undergo treatment if cancer is detected, and ability to cooperate with and tolerate the Pap smear procedure, may obviate the need for cervical cancer screening.	http://www.ahrq.gov/clinic/uspstf/uspscerv.htm

CANCER, CERVICAL						

Disease Screening	Organization	Date	Population	Recommendations	Comments	Source
Cancer, Cervical (continued)	ACS	2007	Women aged ≥ 70 years	Discontinue screening if ≥3 normal Paps in a row and no abnormal Pap in the last 10 years. [e]		http://www.cancer.org
	ACS USPSTF	2007 2003	Women without a cervix	1. Recommends against routine Pap smear screening in women who have had a total hysterectomy for benign disease and no history of abnormal cell growth. 2. Evidence is insufficient to recommend for or against the routine use of new technologies to screen for cervical cancer.		http://www.cancer.org http://www.ahrq.gov/clinic/uspstf/uspscerv.htm

[a]If sexual history is unknown or considered unreliable, screening should begin at age 18 years.
[b]New tests to improve cancer detection include liquid-based/thin-layer preparations, computer-assisted screening methods, and human papillomavirus testing. (Am Fam Phys 2001;64-729)
[c]ACS risk factors include DES exposure before birth, HIV infection, or other forms of immunosuppression, including chronic steroid use.
[d]Most of the benefit can be obtained by beginning screening within 3 years of onset of sexual activity or age 21.
[e]Women with Hx cervical cancer, DES exposure, HIV infection, or weakened immune system should continue to have screening as long as in good health.

Disease Screening	Organization	Date	Population	Recommendations	Comments	Source
CANCER, COLORECTAL						
Cancer, Colorectal	ACG	2005	African Americans, aged ≥ 45 years	Screen with colonoscopy as first-line method.	1. African Americans have a younger mean age of onset of colorectal cancer compared with other groups. 2. African Americans have a greater incidence of cancerous lesions in the proximal large bowel.	Am J Gastroenterol 2005;100:515 http://www.acg.gi.org/physicians/clinicalupdates.asp#guidelines
	AAFP ACS[g] ASGE USMTFCC[a] USPSTF	2007 2007 2006 2003 2002	Age ≥ 50 years at average risk[b]	Screen with 1 of the following strategies[c,d,e]: 1. FOBT annually[f] 2. Flexible sigmoidoscopy every 5 years 3. FOBT annually plus flexible sigmoidoscopy every 5 years[g] 4. Colonoscopy every 10 years[h]	1. The USPSTF "strongly recommends" colorectal cancer screening in this group. 2. Only 35% of women with advanced neoplasia would have had their lesions detected on sigmoidoscopy. (NEJM 2005;352:2061) 3. FOBT alone decreased colorectal cancer mortality by 33% compared with those who were not screened. (Gastroenterology 2004;126) 4. New techniques such as CT virtual colonoscopy (Ann Intern Med 2005;142:635) or fecal DNA (NEJM 2004;351:2704) are not recommended for screening at this time. 5. Sensitivity and specificity for lesions ≥ 10 mm ACBE vs. CT colonoscopy (CTC) vs. colonoscopy for follow-up of GI bleeding were: ACBE (48%; 90%) vs. CTC (59%; 96%) vs. colonoscopy (98%; 99%). (Lancet 2005;365:305)	http://www.aafp.org/online/en/home/clinical/exam.html http://www.cancer.org Gastrointestinal Endoscopy 2006;63:546 Gastroenterology 2003;124:544 http://www.ahrq.gov/clinic/uspstf/uspscolo.htm
	UK-NHS	2007	Adults aged 60–69 years	Program screen every 2 years with fecal occult blood testing.		http://www.cancerscreening.nhs.uk/bowel/index.html
			Adults aged ≥ 70 years	Patient-initiated screening covered by NHS.		

Disease Screening	Organization	Date	Population	Recommendations	Comments	Source
Cancer, Colorectal (continued)	USMTFCC[a]	2003	Persons at increased risk based on family history[i]	*Group I:* Screening colonoscopy at age 40 years, or 10 years younger than the earliest diagnosis in their family, and repeated every 5 years. *Group II:* Follow average risk recommendations, but begin at age 40 years. *Group III:* See Average Risk.		http://www.cancer.org Gastroenterology 2003;124:544

[a]U.S. Multisociety Task Force on Colorectal Cancer (ACG, ACP, AGA, ASGE).

[b]Risk factors indicating need for earlier/more frequent screening: personal history of colorectal cancer or adenomatous polyps or hepatoblastoma, colorectal cancer or polyps in a first-degree relative < 60 years old or in 2 first-degree relatives of any age, personal history of chronic inflammatory bowel disease, and family with hereditary colorectal cancer syndromes. [Ann Intern Med 1998;128(1):900, NEJM 1994;331(25):1669, NEJM 1995;332(13):861] Additional high-risk group: history of ≥ 30 Gy radiation to whole abdomen; all upper abdominal fields; pelvic, thoracic, lumbar, or sacral spine. Begin monitoring 10 years after radiation or at age 35, whichever occurs last. (http://www.survivorshipguidelines.org) Screening colonoscopy in those aged ≥ 80 years results in only 15% of the expected gain in life expectancy in younger patients. (JAMA 2006;295:2357) ACG treats African Americans as high-risk group. See separate recommendation above.

[c]A positive result on an FOBT should be followed by colonoscopy. An alternative is flexible sigmoidoscopy and air-contrast BE.

[d]FOBT should be performed on 2 samples from 3 consecutive specimens obtained at home.

[e]USPSTF did not find direct evidence that screening colonoscopy is effective in reducing colorectal cancer mortality rates.

[f]Use the guaiac-based test with dietary restriction, or an immunochemical test without dietary restriction. Two samples from each of 3 consecutive stools should be examined without rehydration. Rehydration increases the false-positive rate.

[g]ACS prefers option #3 over other strategies.

[h]Population-based retrospective analysis: risk of developing colorectal cancer remains decreased for > 10 years following a negative colonoscopy. (JAMA 2006;295:2366)

[i]*Group I:* First-degree relative with colon cancer or adenomatous polyps at age < 60 years, or 2 first-degree relatives with colorectal cancer at any time. *Group II:* First-degree relative with colorectal cancer or adenomatous polyps at age ≥ 60 years or 2 second-degree relatives with colorectal cancer. *Group III:* 1 second- or third-degree relative with colorectal cancer.

DRE = digital rectal exam; FOBT = fecal occult blood testing

CANCER, ENDOMETRIAL					
Disease Screening	**Organization**	**Date**	**Population**	**Recommendations**	**Comments**	**Source**
Cancer, Endometrial	ACS	2007	All post-menopausal women	Inform women about risks and symptoms of endometrial cancer, and strongly encourage women to report any unexpected bleeding or spotting.	1. *Benefits:* There is inadequate evidence that screening with endometrial sampling or transvaginal ultrasound decreases mortality. *Harms:* Based on solid evidence, screening with transvaginal ultrasound will result in unnecessary additional examinations because of low specificity. Based on solid evidence, endometrial biopsy may result in discomfort, bleeding, infection, and, rarely, uterine perforation. (NCI, 2007) 2. Presence of endometrial cells in Pap test from postmenopausal women not taking exogenous hormones is abnormal and requires further evaluation. Pap test is insensitive for endometrial screening. 3. Endometrial thickness of < 4 mm on transvaginal ultrasound is associated with low risk of endometrial cancer. [Obstet Gynecol 1991;78(2):195] 4. Most cases of endometrial cancer are diagnosed as a result of symptoms reported by patients, and a high proportion of these cases are diagnosed at an early stage and have high rates of survival. (NCI, 2007)	http://www.cancer.org

CANCER, ENDOMETRIAL					
Disease Screening	Organization	Date	Population	Recommendations	Comments	Source
Cancer, Endometrial (continued)	ACS	2007	All women at high risk for endometrial cancer[a]	Annual screening beginning at age 35 years with endometrial biopsy.	1. Variable screening with ultrasound among women (aged 25–65 years; $n = 292$) at high risk for HNPCC mutation detected no cancers from ultrasound. Two endometrial cases occurred in the cohort that presented with symptoms. (Cancer 2002;94:1708) 2. The WHI demonstrated that combined estrogen and progestin did not increase risk of endometrial cancer but did increase rate of endometrial biopsies and ultrasound exams prompted by abnormal uterine bleeding. (JAMA 2003;290)	http://www.cancer.org

[a]High-risk women are those known to carry hereditary nonpolyposis colorectal cancer–associated genetic mutations, or at high risk to carry mutation, or who are from families with suspected autosomal dominant predisposition to colon cancer.
HNPCC = hereditary nonpolyposis colorectal cancer; WHI = Women's Health Initiative

CANCER, GASTRIC

Disease Screening	Organization	Date	Population	Recommendations	Comments	Source
Cancer, Gastric				There are currently no recommendations regarding screening for gastric cancer.	1. Population endoscopic screening for gastric cancer in moderate- to high-risk population subgroups is cost effective (non-U.S. populations). (Clin Gastroenterol Hepatol 2006;4:709) 2. *Benefits:* There is fair evidence that screening would result in no decrease in gastric cancer mortality in the United States. *Harms:* There is good evidence that EGD screening would result in rare but serious side effects, such as perforation, cardiopulmonary events, aspiration pneumonia, and bleeding. (NCI, 2007)	

CANCER, LIVER

Disease Screening	Organization	Date	Population	Recommendations	Comments	Source
Cancer, Liver (Hepatocellular Carcinoma, HCC)	AASLD	2005	Adults at high risk for HCC,[a] including those awaiting liver transplantation	Surveillance with ultrasound every 6–12 months.	1. AFP alone should not be used for screening unless ultrasound is not available. 2. *Benefits:* Based on fair evidence, screening would not result in a decrease in HCC-related mortality. *Harms:* Based on fair evidence, screening would result in rare but serious side effects associated with needle biopsy, such as needle-track seeding, hemorrhage, bile peritonitis, and pneumothorax. (NCI, 2007)	Hepatology 2005;42:1208
	British Society of Gastroenterology	2003	Adults	Surveillance with abdominal ultrasound and AFP every 6 months should be considered for high-risk groups.[b]		Gut 2003;52(Suppl III):iii http://www.bsg.org.uk/

[a] *HBsAg+ persons (carriers):* Asian males ≥ 40 years, Asian females ≥ 50 years; all cirrhotics; family history HCC; Africans > 20 years; *non-hepatitis B carriers:* hepatitis C; alcoholic cirrhosis; genetic hemochromatosis; primary biliary cirrhosis.

[b] All persons with established cirrhosis with HBV, HCV, or hemochromatosis; males with cirrhosis due to alcohol or primary biliary cirrhosis. If surveillance offered, patients should be aware of implications of early diagnosis and lack of proven survival benefit.

Disease Screening	Organization	Date	Population	Recommendations	Comments	Source
CANCER, LUNG						
Cancer, Lung	AAFP USPSTF	2007 2004	Asymptomatic persons	Evidence is insufficient to recommend for or against lung cancer screening.	1. Counsel all patients against tobacco use, even when over 50 years of age. Smokers who quit gain ~10 years of increased life expectancy. (BMJ 2004;328) 2. *Benefits:* Based on fair evidence, screening with sputum or CXR does not reduce mortality from lung cancer. Evidence is inadequate to assess mortality benefit of LDCT. *Harms:* Based on solid evidence, screening would lead to false-positive tests and unnecessary invasive procedures. (CNCI, 2007)	http://www.aafp.org/online/en/home/clinical/exam.html http://www.ahrq.gov/clinic/uspstf/uspslung.htm
	ACCP CTF	2003 2003	Asymptomatic persons	Routine screening for lung cancer with CXR, sputum cytology not recommended. Evidence is insufficient to recommend for or against screening with low-dose CT (LDCT). (ACCP; CTF only)	3. The NCI is conducting the National Lung Screening Test (NLST), an RCT comparing LDCT and CXR for detecting and reducing lung cancer mortality among persons at risk for lung cancer. (http://www.cancer.gov/nlst)	http://www.chestnet.org/education/guidelines/index.php Chest 2003;123:835–885 CA Cancer J Clin 2004;54:41 http://www.ctfphc.org
	ACS	2001	Asymptomatic persons	Guidance in shared decision-making regarding screening of high risk persons.	4. Spiral CT screening can detect greater number of heavy smokers with stage 1 lung cancer. (NEJM 2006;355:1763–1771) 5. Although screening increases the rate of lung cancer diagnosis and treatment, it may not reduce the risk of advanced lung cancer or death from lung cancer. (JAMA 2007;297:995)	http://www.cancer.org

			CANCER, ORAL		
Disease Screening	**Organization**	**Date**	**Population**	**Recommendations**	**Comments**	**Source**
Cancer, Oral	AAFP USPSTF	2007 2004	Asymptomatic persons	Evidence is insufficient to recommend for or against routinely screening adults for oral cancer.	1. Risk factors: regular alcohol or tobacco use. 2. An RCT of visual screening for oral cancer (at 3-year intervals) showed decreased oral cancer mortality among screened males (but not females) who were tobacco and/or alcohol users over an 8-year period. (Lancet 2005;365:1927)	http://www.aafp.org/online/en/home/clinical/exam.html http://www.ahrq.gov/clinic/uspstf/uspsoral.htm
	COG	2006	History of radiation to head, oropharynx, neck, or total body Acute/chronic GVHD	Annual oral cavity exam.		http://www.survivorshipguidelines.org

CANCER, OVARIAN

Disease Screening	Organization	Date	Population	Recommendations	Comments	Source
Cancer, Ovarian	AAFP USPSTF	2007 2004	Asymptomatic women[a]	Recommends against routine screening.	1. Risk factors: aged > 60 years; low parity; personal history of endometrial, colon, or breast cancer; family history of ovarian cancer; and hereditary ovarian cancer syndrome. Use of oral contraceptives decreases risk of ovarian cancer. 2. *Benefit:* There is inadequate evidence to determine whether routine screening for ovarian cancer with serum markers such as CA 125 levels, transvaginal ultrasound, or pelvic examinations would result in a decrease in mortality from ovarian cancer. *Harm:* Based on solid evidence, routine screening for ovarian cancer would result in many diagnostic laparoscopies and laparotomies for each ovarian cancer found. (NCI, 2007)	http://www.aafp.org/online/en/home/clinical/exam.html http://www.ahrq.gov/clinic/uspstf/uspsovar.htm
	AAFP USPSTF	2007 2005	Women whose family history is associated with an increased risk for deleterious mutations in *BRCA1* or *BRCA2* genes[b]	Recommends referral for genetic counseling and evaluation for *BRCA* testing.	3. Preliminary results from the Prostate, Lung, Colorectal and Ovarian (PLCO) Cancer Screening Trial: At the time of baseline exam, positive predictive value for invasive cancer was 3.7% for an abnormal CA 125, 1% for an abnormal transvaginal ultrasound, and 23.5% if both tests were abnormal. (Am J Obstet Gynecol 2005;193:1630)	http://www.aafp.org/online/en/home/clinical/exam.html http://www.ahrq.gov/clinic/uspstf/uspsbrgen.htm

[a]Lifetime risk of ovarian cancer in a woman with no affected relatives is 1 in 70. If 1 first-degree relative has ovarian cancer, lifetime risk is 5%. If 2 or more first-degree relatives have ovarian cancer, lifetime risk is 7%. Women with 2 or more family members affected by ovarian cancer have a 3% chance of having a hereditary ovarian cancer syndrome. These women have a 40% lifetime risk of ovarian cancer.

[b]USPSTF recommends against routine referral for genetic counseling or routine BRCA testing of women whose family history is not associated with increased risk for deleterious mutation in BRCA1 or BRCA2 genes.

CANCER, PANCREATIC					
Disease Screening	**Organization**	**Date**	**Population**	**Recommendations**	**Comments**	**Source**
Cancer, Pancreatic	AAFP USPSTF	2007 2004	Asymptomatic persons	Recommends against routine screening.	1. Cigarette smoking has consistently been associated with increased risk of pancreatic cancer. 2. USPSTF concluded that the harms of screening for pancreatic cancer due to the very low prevalance, limited accuracy of available screening tests, invasive nature of diagnostic tests, and poor outcomes of treatment, exceed any potential benefits.	http://www.aafp.org/online/en/home/clinical/exam.html http://www.ahrq.gov/clinic/uspstf/uspspanc.htm

CANCER, PROSTATE

Disease Screening	Organization	Date	Population	Recommendations	Comments	Source
Cancer, Prostate	ACS	2007	Men aged ≥ 50 years[a]	Offer annual PSA and DRE if ≥ 10-year life expectancy. [b]		http://www.cancer.org
	AAFP USPSTF	2007 2002	Asymptomatic men	Evidence insufficient to recommend for or against routine screening using PSA or DRE.	1. There is good evidence that PSA can detect early-stage prostate cancer, but mixed and inconclusive evidence that early detection improves health outcomes or mortality. 2. *Benefit*: Insufficient evidence to establish whether a decrease in mortality from prostate cancer occurs with screening by DRE or serum PSA. *Harm*: Based on good evidence, screening with PSA and/or DRE detects some prostate cancers that would never have caused important clinical problems. Based on good evidence, current prostate cancer treatments result in permanent side effects in many men, including erectile dysfunction and urinary incontinence. (NCI, 2007) 3. Further evaluation is recommended when PSA > 4. However, a study found an overall prevalence of prostate cancer of 15% in men with a PSA < 4. (NEJM 2004;350) 4. Men with localized, low-grade prostate cancers (Gleason score 2–4) have a minimal risk of dying from prostate cancer during 20 years of follow-up (6 deaths per 1,000 person-years). (JAMA 2005;293:2095)	http://www.aafp.org/online/en/home/clinical/exam.html http://www.ahrq.gov/clinic/uspstf/uspsprca.htm

				CANCER, PROSTATE		
Disease Screening	**Organization**	**Date**	**Population**	**Recommendations**	**Comments**	**Source**
Cancer, Prostate (continued)					5. Radical prostatectomy (vs. watchful waiting) reduces disease-specific and overall mortality in patients with symptomatic early prostate cancer. (NEJM 2005;352:1977) Whether this benefit translates to asymptomatic patients identified through screening measures is unknown. 6. PSA rise of > 2 per year is associated with recurrence and death. (NEJM 2004;351) It is not known if using PSA velocity to determine treatment is useful.	
	UK-NHS	2007	Asymptomatic men	Informed decision making.	See informational leaflet at: http://www.cancerscreening.nhs.uk/prostate/prostate-patient-info-sheet.pdf	www.cancerscreening.nhs.uk

[a]Men in high-risk groups (one or more first-degree relatives diagnosed before age 65, African Americans) should begin screening at age 45. Men at higher risk due to multiple first-degree relatives affected at an early age could begin testing at age 40. (http://www.cancer.org/)
[b]Men who ask their doctor to make the decision should be tested. Discouraging testing is not appropriate, nor is not offering testing.

| | CANCER, SKIN | | | | | |

Disease Screening	Organization	Date	Population	Recommendations	Comments	Source
Cancer, Skin (melanoma)	AAFP USPSTF	2007 2001	Asymptomatic persons	Evidence is insufficient to recommend for or against routine screening using a total-body skin examination for early detection of cutaneous melanoma, basal cell carcinoma, or squamous cell skin cancer. [a,b]	1. *Benefits:* Evidence is inadequate to determine whether visual examination of the skin in asymptomatic individuals would lead to a reduction in mortality from melanomatous skin cancer. *Harms:* Based on fair though unqualified evidence, visual examination of the skin in asymptomatic persons may lead to unavoidable increases in harmful consequences. (NCI, 2007) 2. American Academy of Dermatology opposes indoor tanning and suggests a ban on production and sale of indoor tanning equipment. (2004) (http://www.aad.org)	http://www.aafp.org/online/en/home/clinical/exam.html http://www.ahrq.gov/clinic/uspstf/uspsskca.htm

[a]Clinicians should remain alert for skin lesions with malignant features when examining patients for other reasons, particularly patients with established risk factors. Risk factors for skin cancer include: evidence of melanocytic precursors, large numbers of common moles, immunosuppression, any history of radiation, family or personal history of skin cancer, substantial cumulative lifetime sun exposure, intermittent intense sun exposure or severe sunburns in childhood, freckles, poor tanning ability, and light skin, hair, and eye color.

[b]Consider educating patients with established risk factors for skin cancer (see above) concerning signs and symptoms suggesting skin cancer and the possible benefits of periodic self-exam. (USPSTF) (ACS) (COG)

CANCER, TESTICULAR

Disease Screening	Organization	Date	Population	Recommendations	Comments	Source
Cancer, Testicular	AAFP USPSTF	2007 2004	Asymptomatic adolescent and adult males[a]	Recommend against routine screening.	1. *Benefits:* Based on fair evidence, screening would not result in appreciable decrease in mortality, in part because therapy at each stage is so effective. *Harm:* Based on fair evidence, screening would result in unnecessary diagnostic procedures. (NCI, 2007)	http://aafp.org/online/en/ home/clinical/exam.htm http://www.ahrq.gov/clinic/ uspstf/uspstest.htm
	ACS	2004	Asymptomatic men	Testicular exam by physician as part of routine cancer-related check-up.		http://www.cancer.org

[a] Patients with history of cryptorchidism, orchiopexy, family history of testicular cancer, or testicular atrophy should be informed of their increased risk for developing testicular cancer and counseled about screening. Such patients may then elect to be screened or to perform testicular self-exam. Adolescent and young adult males should be advised to seek prompt medical attention if they notice a scrotal abnormality. (USPSTF)

CANCER, THYROID						

Disease Screening	Organization	Date	Population	Recommendations	Comments	Source
Cancer, Thyroid	AAFP	2007	Asymptomatic persons	Recommends against the use of ultrasound screening in asymptomatic persons.	1. Neck palpation for nodules in asymptomatic individuals has sensitivity 15%–38%; specificity 93%–100%. Only a small proportion of nodular thyroid glands are neoplastic, resulting in a high false-positive rate. (USPSTF)	http://www.aafp.org/online/en/home/clinical/exam.html

CAROTID ARTERY STENOSIS					
Disease Screening	Organization	Date	Population	Recommendations	Comments	Source

Disease Screening	Organization	Date	Population	Recommendations	Comments	Source
Carotid Artery Stenosis (asymptomatic)	ASN	2007	Asymptomatic adults	Screening of the general population or a selected population based on age, gender, or any other variable alone is not recommended.	1. The prevalence of internal carotid artery stenosis (ICAS) of ≥ 70% is low in persons with only atherosclerosis risk factors (1.8%–2.3%), intermediate in those with angina or MI (3.1%), and highest in those with PAD (12.5%) or AAA (8.8%). Advanced age (> 54 years) and lower diastolic BP (< 83 mm Hg) increased prevalence of ICAS. (J Vasc Surg 2003;37:1226–1233) 2. Asymptomatic Carotid Surgery Trial (ACST) (Lancet 2004;363:1491): The absolute risk reduction for stroke or death at 5 years was 5.4%, with significant benefit observed in women (4% absolute risk reduction) as well as in men (8.2% risk reduction). 3. Severe CAS and coexisting conditions: carotid stenting with use of emboli-protection device is *not* inferior to CEA. [NEJM 2004 Oct 7;351(15):1493–1501]	J Neuroimaging 2007;17:19–47

CHLAMYDIAL INFECTION						
Disease Screening	Organization	Date	Population	Recommendations	Comments	Source
Chlamydial Infection	USPSTF	2007	Women aged ≤ 24 years who are sexually active, and older non-pregnant women at increased risk[a]	Recommends at least annual screening; optimal interval for screening is uncertain.[b]	1. Antigen detection tests, nonamplified nucleic acid hybridization, and amplified DNA assays may provide improved sensitivity, lower expense, availability, and/or timeliness of results over culture. 2. Noninvasive methods such as urine specimens and vaginal swabs appear reliable. 3. Early detection and treatment of women at risk for chlamydial infection (prevalence 7%) reduced the incidence of pelvic inflammatory disease from 28 per 1,000 woman-years to 13 per 1,000 woman-years.	http://www.ahrq.gov/clinic/uspstf/uspschlm.htm
	USPSTF	2007	Pregnant women aged < 24 years, and older pregnant women at increased risk	Screen during first trimester or first prenatal visit.	4. Recent population-based studies show overall prevalence of chlamydial infection in persons aged 18–26 years to be 4.7%, with rates six-fold higher among African Americans. Prevalence rates in men were 3.5%. (JAMA 2004;291:2229) 5. Prevalence of asymptomatic chlamydial infection among military recruits age 18–25 was 8.5%. (South Med J 2007;100:478)	

CHLAMYDIAL INFECTION

Disease Screening	Organization	Date	Population	Recommendations	Comments	Source
Chlamydial Infection (continued)	USPSTF	2007	Women aged ≥ 25 years	Recommends against routinely screening women aged ≥ 25 years, whether or not they are pregnant, if they are not at increased risk.		
	USPSTF	2007	Men	Evidence insufficient to assess the balance of benefits to harms of screening.		

[a]Aged ≤ 25 years, new male sex partners or 2 or more partners during preceding year, inconsistent use of barrier methods, history of prior STD, African-American race, cervical ectopy.
[b]For women with a previous negative screening test, the interval for rescreening should take into account changes in sexual partners. If there is evidence that a woman is at low risk for infection (eg, in a mutually monogamous relationship with a previous history of negative screening tests for chlamydial infection), it may not be necessary to screen frequently. Rescreening at 6 to 12 months may be appropriate for previously infected women because of high rates of reinfection. USPSTF (2005) also recommends screening all high-risk sexually active women for gonorrheal infection.

CHOLESTEROL & LIPID DISORDERS

Disease Screening	Organization	Date	Population	Recommendations	Comments	Source
Cholesterol & Lipid Disorders	USPSTF	2007	Infants, children, adolescents, or young adults (aged < 20 years)	Insufficient evidence to recommend for or against routine screening.[a]	1. Effectiveness of treatment interventions in children with dyslipidemia remains a critical research gap. 2. Age to stop screening is not established. Clinical trial data demonstrate that persons older than 65 years of age derive the same benefit from cholesterol reduction as younger adults. 3. Base treatment decisions on at least 2 cholesterol levels. 4. Intensive lipid-modulating therapy (LDL < 60 mg/dL; increase in HDL ≥ 15 mg/dL) is associated with plaque and atheroma volume regression (the ASTEROID trial). (JAMA 2006;295:1556)	http://www.ahrq.gov/clinic/uspstf/uspschlip.htm Pediatrics 2007;120:e189–e214
	NCEP III	2004	Men and women aged > 20 years	Check fasting lipoprotein panel (if testing opportunity is nonfasting, use nonfasting TC and HDL) every 5 years if in desirable range; otherwise see management algorithm.[b]		Circulation 2002;106:3143–3421 Circulation 2004;110:227–239 http://www.nhlbi.nih.gov/guidelines/cholesterol/atp3upd04.htm

				CHOLESTEROL & LIPID DISORDERS		
Disease Screening	Organization	Date	Population	Recommendations	Comments	Source
Cholesterol & Lipid Disorders (continued)	AAFP USPSTF	2006 2001	Men aged 20–35 years Women aged 20–45 years	Recommends routine screening of individuals with major CHD risk factors.[c] Optimal screening interval uncertain. Makes no recommendation for or against routine screening for lipid disorders in the absence of known CHD risk factors.		http://www.aafp.org/exam http://www.ahrq.gov/clinic/ uspstf/uspschol.htm
	AAFP USPSTF	2007 2001	Men aged ≥ 35 years Women aged ≥ 45 years	Strongly recommends routine screening for lipid disorders and treatment of abnormal lipid in people who are at increased risk of CHD.[c] Random total cholesterol and HDL, cholesterol or fasting lipid profile, periodicity based on risk factors.		Am J Prev Med 2001;20(35):73–76 http://www.aafp.org/exam/ Geriatrics 2003;58:33–38 http://www.ahrq.gov/clinic/ uspstf/uspschol.htm

[a]AHA: Low efficacy of targeted screening of children based on family history. Sensitivity and specificity of screening complicated by variability in total cholesterol and HDL based on race, gender, and sexual maturation. (Circulation 2007;115:1948-1967)

[b]Classify fasting TC < 200 mg/dL as desirable, 200–239 mg/dL as borderline, or ≥ 240 mg/dL as high. Classify HDL < 40 as low, and ≥ 60 as high. Classify LDL < 100 as optimal, 100–129 as near or above optimal, 130–159 as borderline high, 160–189 as high, and ≥ 190 as very high. If TC < 200 mg/dL and HDL ≥ 40 mg/dL, then repeat in 5 years; if non-fasting TC ≥ 200 mg/dL or HDL < 40 mg/dL, then check fasting lipids and risk stratify based on LDL (see Management algorithm). Advanced lipoprotein testing does not predict carotid intima-media thickness better than traditionally measured lipid values. (Ann Intern Med 2005;142:742–750)

[c]Hypertension, smoking, diabetes, family history of CHD before age 50 (male relatives) or age 60 (female relatives), family history suggestive of familial hyperlipidemia.

	CORONARY ARTERY DISEASE				
Disease Screening	Organization	Date	Population	Recommendations	Comments	Source
Coronary Artery Disease	AAFP AHA USPSTF	2007 2007 2004	Adults at low risk of CHD events[a]	Recommends *against* routine screening with resting ECG, ETT, or electron-beam CT for coronary calcium.[b]	1. Key questions to answer in RCT are (1) effect of testing asymptomatic person on subsequent CHD morbidity and mortality; (2) effect in women; (3) cost-effectiveness. 2. Specific recommendations regarding non-invasive testing in the evaluation of women with suspected CAD have also been published. (Circulation 2005;111:682–696)	http://www.aafp.org/online/en/home/clinical/exam.html http://www.ahrq.gov/clinic/uspstf/uspsacad.htm Ann Intern Med 2004;140:569 Circulation 2005;112:771–776 Circulation 2007;115:402-426
	AHA	2007	Adults at intermediate risk of CHD events	May be reasonable to consider use of coronary artery calcium measurement.[b]		Circulation 2007;115:402-426
	AAFP AHA USPSTF	2007 2007 2004	Adults at high risk of CHD events[a]	Insufficient evidence to recommend for or against routine screening with ECG, ETT, or electron-beam CT for coronary calcium.[b]		Ann Intern Med 2004;140:569 http://www.aafp.org/online/en/home/clinical/exam.html http://www.ahrq.gov/clinic/uspstf/uspsacad.htm Circulation 2005;112:771–776

CORONARY ARTERY DISEASE						
Disease Screening	Organization	Date	Population	Recommendations	Comments	Source
Coronary Artery Disease (continued)	Third Joint Task Force of European and other Societies on Cardiovascular Disease Prevention	2003	Age ≥ 40	Estimate risk based on the SCORE (Systematic Coronary Risk Evaluation) system.[b]		http://www.escardio.org/ initiatives/prevention/ prevention-tools/SCORE-Risk-Charts.htm European J Cardiovascular Prevention and Rehab. 2003; 10(Suppl 1): S1–S78

[a]Increased risk for CHD events: older age, male gender, high blood pressure, smoking, elevated lipid levels, diabetes, obesity, sedentary lifestyle. Risk assessment tool for estimating 10-year risk of developing CHD events available online or see Appendix V. (http://hp2010.nhlbihin.net/atpiii/calculator.asp)

[b]AHA scientific statement (2006): Asymptomatic persons should be assessed for CHD risk. Individuals found to be at low risk (< 10% 10-year risk) or at high risk (> 20% 10-year risk) do not benefit from coronary calcium assessment. High-risk individuals are already candidates for intensive risk reducing therapies. In clinically selected, intermediate-risk patients, it may be reasonable to use EBCT or MDCT to refine clinical risk prediction and select patients for more aggressive target values for lipid-lowering therapies. (Circulation 2006;114:1761–1791)

DEMENTIA

Disease Screening	Organization	Date	Population	Recommendations	Comments	Source
Dementia	AAN USPSTF	2004 2003	Elderly, asymptomatic	Insufficient evidence to recommend for or against routine screening for dementia.	1. Screening instruments are useful for detecting multiple cognitive deficits and determining a baseline for future assessments.[b] 2. Short Test of Mental Status (STMS) slightly more effective than Mini Mental State Examination (MMSE) in differentiating between cognitively healthy and MCI (Arch Neurol 2003;60:1777–1781)	Ann Intern Med 2003;138:925–926 Ann Intern Med 2003;138:927–937 Neurology 2001;56:1133–1142 Neurology 2001;56:1143–1153 http://www.ahrq.gov/clinic/uspstf/uspsdeme.htm
	AAN AGS	2003 2003	Elderly, mild cognitive impairment (MCI)[a]	Persons with MCI should be evaluated regularly for progression to dementia. (Review of MCI: Lancet 2006;367(9518):1262)	3. Reversible causes of dementia include vitamin B_{12} deficiency, neurosyphilis, and hypothyroidism. Be aware of other causes of mental status changes, such as depression, delirium, medication effects, and coexisting illnesses. 4. Homocysteine lowering with B vitamins and folate does not improve cognitive performance in healthy older adults. (NEJM 2006;354: 2764)	http://www.aan.com/professionals http://www.americangeriatrics.org Neurology 2001;56:1133–1142 Mini Mental State Exam: J Psychiatr Res 1975;12:189, also see Mini Mental State Examination in Appendix I Short Test of Mental Status: Mayo Clinic Proc 1987;62:281–288

[a]Triggers that should initiate an assessment for dementia include difficulties in (1) learning and retaining new information, (2) handling complex tasks (eg, balancing a checkbook or cooking a meal), (3) reasoning ability (eg, a new disregard for social norms), (4) spatial ability and orientation (eg, difficulty driving, or getting lost), (5) language (eg, difficulties in word-finding), and (6) behavior (eg, appearing more passive or more irritable than usual). DSM-IV diagnosis of dementia requires: (1) evidence of decline in functional abilities and (2) evidence of multiple cognitive deficiencies. MCI criteria: memory complaint, preferably corroborated by an informant; objective memory impairment; normal general cognitive function; intact activities of daily living; not demented. 6%–25% of MCI patients progress to dementia each year.

[b]Articles comparing validated cognitive impairment screening instruments: J Neurol Neurosurg Psychiatry 2007;78:790–799. JAMA 2007;297:2391–2404.

Note: American Academy of Neurology website includes an "AAN Encounter Kit for Dementia," a web-based algorithm to assist coding, diagnosis, and pharmacologic management of cognitive disorders in adults (MCI and dementia). (http://aan.com/go/practice/quality/dementia)

Disease Screening	Organization	Date	Population	Recommendations	Comments	Source
Depression	AAFP CTF USPSTF[a]	2007 2005 2002	Children and adolescents	Insufficient evidence to recommend for or against routine screening.	1. Clues to depression include poor school performance, alcohol or drug use, and deteriorating parental or peer relationships. 2. Clues to suicide risk include family dysfunction, physical and sexual abuse, substance abuse, history of recurrent or severe depression, and prior suicide attempt or plans.[b]	http://aafp.org/online/ en/home/clinical/ exam.html CMAJ 2005;172:33 http://ahrq.gov/clinic/ uspstf/uspsdepr.htm
	NICE	2005	Children and young adults (aged 5–18 years)	Healthcare professionals in primary care, schools, and other relevant community settings should be trained to detect symptoms of depression, and to assess children and young adults who may be at risk for depression.		http://guidance.nice. org.uk/CG28
	Bright Futures	2002	Adolescents	Annual screening for behaviors or emotions that might indicate depression or risk of suicide.		http://brightfutures. aap.org/web/

Disease Screening	Organization	Date	Population	Recommendations	Comments	Source
Depression (continued)	AAFP USPSTF[a]	2007 2002	Adults	Recommend screening adults for depression in practices with systems in place to assure accurate diagnosis, effective treatment, and follow-up.	1. See screening instruments [Geriatric Depression Scale, Beck Depression Inventory (Short Form), PRIME-MD; PHQ-9] in Appendix I. 2. Optimal screening interval is unknown.	http://aafp.org/online/en/home/clinical/exam.html http://ahrq.gov/clinic/uspstf/uspsdepr.htm
	NICE	2004	High-risk groups[c]	Recommend screening in primary care and general hospital settings.		http://www.nice.org.uk/CG23/

[a]Update in progress.
[b]Suicide risk increases as the number of conditions increases. Parents of adolescents at risk for suicide should reduce access to firearms, weapons, or potentially lethal drugs in the home.
[c]High-risk groups: past history of depression, significant physical illness causing disability, other mental health problems such as dementia.

DEVELOPMENTAL DYSPLASIA OF THE HIP

Disease Screening	Organization	Date	Population	Recommendations	Comments	Source
Developmental Dysplasia of the Hip (DDH)	USPSTF	2006	Infants	Evidence is insufficient to recommend routine screening for developmental dysplasia of the hip in infants as a means to prevent adverse outcomes.	1. There is evidence that screening leads to earlier identification; however 60%–80% of the hips of newborns identified as abnormal or suspicious for DDH by physician examination and > 90% of those identified by ultrasound in the newborn period resolve spontaneously, requiring no intervention. 2. The USPSTF was unable to assess the balance of benefits and harms of screening for DDH but was concerned about the potential harms associated with treatment, both surgical and non-surgical, of infants identified by routine screening.	http://www.ahrq.gov/clinic/uspstf/uspshipd.htm

DIABETES MELLITUS, GESTATIONAL					
Disease Screening	**Organization**	**Date**	**Population**	**Recommendations**	**Comments**	**Source**
Diabetes Mellitus, Gestational (GDM)	AAFP USPSTF	2007 2003	Asymptomatic pregnant women	Evidence is insufficient to recommend for or against routine screening.	1. High-quality evidence that screening (vs. testing women with symptoms) for GDM reduces important adverse health outcomes for mothers or their infants is lacking. 2. Fasting plasma glucose ≥ 126 mg/dL or a casual plasma glucose ≥ 200 mg/dL meets threshold for diabetes diagnosis, if confirmed on a subsequent day, *and precludes the need for glucose challenge*. (ADA)	http://www.aafp.org/ online/en/home/ clinical/exam.html http://www.ahrq.gov/ clinic/uspstf/uspsgdm. htm
	ADA	2007	Pregnant women	Risk assess all women at first prenatal visit. If clinical characteristics consistent with a *high risk* of GDM,[a] do glucose testing as soon as possible. If no GDM at initial testing,[b] retest between 24 and 28 weeks' gestation. *Average-risk women:* test at 24–28 weeks' gestation. *Low-risk women[c]:* no glucose testing.		Diabetes Care 2007;30(Suppl 1) http://www.diabetes. org/for-health-professionals-and-scientists/cpr.jsp

[a]High risk is defined as (1) obesity (BMI > 27 kg/m²) (see BMI Conversion Table in Appendix IV), (2) strong family history of diabetes, (3) personal history of GDM, (4) glycosuria, (5) previous delivery of large-for-gestational-age infant, or (6) polycystic ovarian syndrome.

[b]Use 1 of 2 approaches to assess: (1) Screen with 50-g oral glucose load. If 1 hour ≥ 130 mg/dL, perform diagnostic 100-g OGTT or (2) diagnostic 100-g OGTT (positive test meets ≥ 2 of: ≥ 95 mg/dL, fasting; ≥ 180 mg/dL at 1 hour, ≥ 155 mg/dL at 2 hours, and ≥ 140 mg/dL at 3 hours).

[c]Low risk for GDM (may *not* need lab screening): < 25 years old; not of Hispanic, African, Native American, South or East Asian, or Pacific Islands ancestry; weight normal before pregnancy; no history of abnormal glucose tolerance; no previous history of poor obstetric outcome; no known diabetes in first-degree relative.

DIABETES MELLITUS, TYPE 2						
Disease Screening	**Organization**	**Date**	**Population**	**Recommendations**	**Comments**	**Source**
Diabetes Mellitus, Type 2	ADA	2007	Children	Fasting plasma glucose at age 10 years or onset of puberty, and every 2 years if overweight (BMI > 85th percentile for age and sex) plus 2 additional risk factors.[a]	1. Fasting plasma glucose is the preferred test in children and nonpregnant adults. Use of A1C for the diagnosis of diabetes is not recommended. (ADA) 2. Cost effectiveness analysis suggests that universal screening is very costly ($360,966 per QALY), in contrast to targeted screening of hypertensives ($34,375 per QALY). (Ann Intern Med 2004;140:689)	Diabetes Care 2007;30 (Suppl 1) http://www.diabetes.org/for-health-professionals-and-scientists/cpr.jsp
	ADA	2007	Adults	Consider screening with fasting glucose or glucose tolerance test at 3-year intervals beginning at age 45, especially if BMI ≥ 25 kg/m²; consider testing earlier or more frequently in overweight patients if diabetes risk factors present.[b]		Diabetes Care 2007;30 (Suppl 1) http://www.diabetes.org/for-health-professionals-and-scientists/cpr.jsp

Disease Screening	Organization	Date	Population	Recommendations	Comments	Source
DIABETES MELLITUS, TYPE 2						
Diabetes Mellitus, Type 2 (continued)	AAFP USPSTF	2007 2003	Adults	Evidence is insufficient to recommend for or against routinely screening asymptomatic adults for type 2 diabetes, impaired glucose tolerance, or impaired fasting glucose.	3. Diagnostic criteria: *Diabetes* = fasting plasma glucose ≥ 126 mg/dL **or** plasma glucose 2 hours after 75 g glucose load ≥ 200 mg/dL *Impaired glucose tolerance* = fasting plasma glucose ≥ 126 mg/dL **and** plasma glucose 2 hours after 75 g glucose load 140–200 mg/dL *Impaired fasting glucose* = fasting plasma glucose 110–125 mg/dL **and** (if measured) plasma glucose 2 hours after 75 g glucose load < 140 mg/dL 4. It has not been demonstrated that beginning diabetes control early as a result of screening provides an incremental benefit compared with initiating treatment after clinical diagnosis. (USPSTF)	http://www.aafp.org/online/en/home/clinical/exam.html http://www.ahrq.gov/clinic/uspstf/uspsdiab.htm

Disease Screening	Organization	Date	Population	Recommendations	Comments	Source
Diabetes Mellitus, Type 2 (continued)	ESC EASD	2007	Adults	Primary screening using a non-invasive risk score, subsequently combined with diagnostic oral glucose tolerance testing in people with high score values.	5. In hypertensives, there is strong evidence that more aggressive blood pressure control is beneficial when diabetes is present. 6. In hypertlipidemia, NCEP III recommends different treatment thresholds and targets when diabetes is present.	http://www.escardio.org/knowledge/guidelines/Guidelines_list.htm?hit=quick
	AAFP USPSTF	2007 2003	Hypertensive or hyperlipidemic adults	Recommends screening for type 2 diabetes (test and frequency not known).		http://www.aafp.org/online/en/home/clinical/exam.html

[a]Risk factors (in addition to overweight): family history of type 2 diabetes in first- or second-degree relative; race/ethnicity (Native American, African American, Latino, Asian American, Pacific Islander); signs of or conditions associated with insulin resistance (acanthosis nigricans, hypertension, dyslipidemia, or polycystic ovary syndrome).

[b]Risk factors (in addition to age ≥ 45 years) include (1) family history of diabetes in parents or siblings; (2) membership in one of the following ethnic groups: African American, Latino, Native American, Asian American, or Pacific Islander; (3) history of impaired fasting glucose, impaired glucose tolerance, gestational diabetes, or mother with infant birthweight > 9 lb; (4) comorbid conditions, including hypertension (> 140/90 mm Hg) or dyslipidemia (HDL < 35 mg/dL or TGs > 250 mg/dL); (5) overweight (BMI ≥ 25 kg/m²); (6) polycystic ovary syndrome or acanthosis nigricans; (7) history of vascular disease; and (8) habitually physically inactive. Diabetes risk calculator available on ADA website. (http://www.diabetes.org/diabetesphd)

FALLS IN THE ELDERLY

Disease Screening	Organization	Date	Population	Recommendations	Comments	Source
Falls in the Elderly	AAOS AGS British Geriatrics Society	2001	All older persons	Ask at least yearly about falls.[a,b]	1. See also page 93 for fall prevention and Appendix II.	JAGS 2001;49:664–672 http://www.american geriatrics.org/products/ positionpapers/falls.pdf http://www.bgs.org.uk/
	CTF	2005	All persons admitted to long-term care facilities	Recommend programs that target the broad range of environmental and resident-specific risk factors to prevent falls and hip fractures.[c]		http://www.ctfphc.org

[a]All who report a single fall should be observed as they stand up from a chair without using their arms, walk several paces, and return (see Appendix II). Those demonstrating no difficulty or unsteadiness need no further assessment. Those who have difficulty or demonstrate unsteadiness, have ≥ 1 fall, or present for medical attention after a fall should have a fall evaluation (see Fall Prevention, page 93).

[b]Risk factors: Intrinsic: lower extremity weakness, poor grip strength, balance disorders, functional and cognitive impairment, visual deficits. Extrinsic: polypharmacy (≥ 4 prescription medications), environment (poor lighting, loose carpets, lack of bathroom safety equipment).

[c]Post-fall assessments may detect previously unrecognized health concerns.

	FAMILY VIOLENCE & ABUSE				
Disease Screening	**Organization**	**Date**	**Population**	**Recommendations**	**Comments**	**Source**

Disease Screening	Organization	Date	Population	Recommendations	Comments	Source
Family Violence & Abuse	AAFP USPSTF	2007 2004	Children, women, and older adults	Insufficient evidence to recommend for or against routine screening of parents or guardians for the physical abuse or neglect of children, of women for intimate partner violence, or of older adults or their caregivers for elder abuse.	1. By law, child abuse must be reported to authorities in all 50 states. 2. Assess adolescents without parent/partner in room. 3. All providers should be aware of physical and behavioral signs and symptoms associated with abuse and neglect, including burns, bruises, and repeated suspect trauma. 4. See also AAP position statement, "The Evaluation of Sexual Abuse in Children." (Pediatrics 2005;116:506) 5. Direct questions should be asked. 6. Inform patient about limits of practitioner/patient confidentiality related to intimate partner violence prior to assessing. 7. Use a private room. 8. If interpreter used, he or she should not be an acquaintance or family relative. Never use children as interpreters. 9. Controversy exists regarding the overall benefit of mandatory reporting of domestic violence. (JAMA 1995;273:1781) 10. Prevalence of domestic violence among women seeking emergency department care was 26% in an urban ED and 21% in a suburban ED. (Arch Intern Med 2006;166:1107) 11. Some states have mandatory reporting of elder abuse and neglect.	http://www.aafp.org/online/en/home/clinical/exam.html http://www.ahrq.gov/clinic/uspstf/uspsfamv.htm
	Family Violence Prevention Fund	2004	Children and adolescents	1) Assess caregivers/parents who accompany their children during new patient visits, at least once per year at well child visits, and thereafter whenever they disclose a new intimate relationship. 2) Assess adolescents during new patient visits, at least once per year at wellness visits, and thereafter whenever they disclose a new intimate relationship.		http://endabuse.org/

FAMILY VIOLENCE & ABUSE

Disease Screening	Organization	Date	Population	Recommendations	Comments	Source
Family Violence & Abuse (continued)				3) Ask whenever signs or symptoms raise concerns. [a]		

[a] Concerns exist when the child or adolescent has obvious physical signs of physical or sexual abuse; behavioral or emotional problems, such as increased aggression, increased fear or anxiety, difficulty sleeping or eating, or other signs of emotional distress; or chronic somatic complaints, or when adults present with obvious physical injuries or history of intimate partner abuse.

GONORRHEA, ASYMPTOMATIC INFECTION

Disease Screening	Organization	Date	Population	Recommendations	Comments	Source
Gonorrhea, Asymptomatic Infection	AAFP USPSTF	2007 2005	Sexually active women	Screen if at increased risk for infection.[a,b]	1. Vaginal culture remains an accurate screening test when transport is suitable. 2. Newer tests, such as nucleic acid amplification and nucleic acid hybridization, have showed improved sensitivity compared with vaginal culture. 3. First-line treatment with fluoroquinolones is no longer recommended due to increased levels of resistance. (http://www.cdc.gov/std/gonorrhea/arg/)	http://www.aafp.org/online/en/home/clinical/exam.html http://www.ahrq.gov/clinic/uspstf/uspsgono.htm
	AAFP USPSTF	2007 2005	Pregnant women	Screen at first prenatal visit if at increased risk for infection.[a,b,c]		
	AAFP USPSTF	2007 2005	Sexually active men	Insufficient evidence to recommend for or against routine screening in men at increased risk for infection.[d]		

[a]Highest risk exists for sexually active women <25 years age. Additional risk factors include history of prior gonorrhea infection, other sexually transmitted infections, new or multiple sexual partners, inconsistent condom use, sex work, and drug use.

[b]In communities with a high prevalence of gonorrhea, broader screening of sexually active young people may be warranted.

[c]If continued risk, or for those who acquired new risk factors during pregnancy, a second screening should be conducted in 3rd trimester.

[d]Primarily due to low prevalence of *asymptomatic* infection in men.

HEARING IMPAIRMENT

Disease Screening	Organization	Date	Population	Recommendations	Comments	Source
Hearing Impairment	Joint Committee on Infant Hearing[a] AAP Bright Futures	2007 2002 2000	Infants	The hearing of all infants should be screened using objective, physiologic measures to identify those with congenital or neonatal-onset hearing loss.	1. Audiologic evaluations should be in progress before 3 months of age. 2. Infants with confirmed hearing loss should receive intervention before 6 months of age. 3. The efficacy of universal newborn hearing screening to improve long-term language outcomes remains uncertain. (JAMA 2001;286: 2000–2010)	Pediatrics 2000;106(4): 798–817 http://www.aap.org http://www.jcih.org
	AAFP USPSTF	2007 2001	Newborns	Insufficient evidence to recommend for or against routine screening of newborns for hearing loss during the post-partum hospitalization.		http://www.aafp.org/ online/en/home/clinical/ exam.html http://www.ahrq.gov/ clinic/uspstf/uspsnbhr. htm
	AAP Bright Futures Joint Committee on Infant Hearing[a]	2003 2002 2000	High-risk infants and children[b,c]	Infants should be screened no later than 3 months of age. Screen infants and children < 2 years of age with increased risk. Screen every 6 months until 3 years of age and at appropriate intervals thereafter if there is risk for delayed-onset hearing loss.		Pediatrics 2000;106(4): 798–817 http://www.aap.org Pediatrics 2003;111: 436–440 http://www.jcih.org
	AAP	2003	High-risk children[c]	Children with frequent recurrent otitis media or middle-ear effusion, or both, should have audiology screening and monitoring of communication skills development.		http://www.aap.org Pediatrics 2003;111: 436–440

HEARING IMPAIRMENT

Disease Screening	Organization	Date	Population	Recommendations	Comments	Source
Hearing Impairment (continued)	AAFP AGS	2007 1997	Adults	Question older adults periodically about hearing impairment, counsel about availability of hearing-aid devices, and make referrals for abnormalities when appropriate.[d,e]		http://www.aafp.org/online/en/home/clinical/exam.html J Am Geriatr Soc 1997; 45:344

[a] Joint Committee on Infant Hearing member organizations: American Academy of Audiology; American Academy of Otolaryngology–Head and Neck Surgery; American Academy of Pediatrics; American Speech-Language-Hearing Association; Council on Education of the Deaf; and Directors of Speech and Hearing Programs in State Health and Welfare Agencies.

[b] Increased neonatal risk: family history of hereditary sensorineural hearing loss, intrauterine infection, craniofacial anomalies, birthweight < 1,500 g, hyperbilirubinemia requiring exchange transfusions, ototoxic medications, bacterial meningitis, Apgar scores 0–4 and 0–6, mechanical ventilation lasting > 5 days, and stigmata associated with a syndrome known to include hearing loss.

[c] Increased childhood risk: patient/caregiver concern regarding hearing, speech, language, or developmental delay; bacterial meningitis; head trauma associated with loss of consciousness or skull fracture; stigmata associated with a syndrome known to include hearing loss; ototoxic medications; recurrent or persistent otitis media with effusion; disorders affecting eustachian tube function; neurofibromatosis type 2; and neurodegenerative disorders. Delayed-onset hearing loss: as above for increased childhood risk plus family history of hereditary childhood hearing loss and intrauterine infection.

[d] See also Appendix II: Functional Assessment Screening in the Elderly.

[e] Review of accuracy and precision of bedside clinical maneuvers for diagnosing hearing impairment: elderly individuals who acknowledge they have hearing impairment require audiometry. Those who do not should be screened with whispered voice test. If passed, no further testing. Those unable to perceive whispered voice require audiometry. The Weber and Rinne tests should not be used for general screening. (JAMA 2006;295:416)

Disease Screening	Organization	Date	Population	Recommendations	Comments	Source
HEMOCHROMATOSIS						
Hemochromatosis (hereditary)	AAFP USPSTF	2007 2006	Asymptomatic adults	Recommends against routine genetic screening for hemochromatosis.	1. There is fair evidence that disease due to hereditary hemochromatosis is rare in the general population. 2. There is poor evidence that early therapeutic phlebotomy improves morbidity and mortality in screening-detected vs. clinically-detected individuals.	http://www.aafp.org/online/en/home/clinical/exam.html http://www.ahrq.gov/clinic/uspstf/uspshemoch.htm
	ACP	2005	Adults	Insufficient evidence to recommend for or against screening.[a] For clinicians who choose to screen, one-time screening of non-Hispanic white men with serum ferritin level and transferrin saturation has highest yield. In case-finding for hereditary hemochromatosis, serum ferritin and transferrin saturation tests should be performed.	If testing performed, cut-off values for serum ferritin level > 200 µg/L in women and > 300 µg/L in men and transferrin saturation > 55% may be used as criteria for case finding, but no general agreement about diagnostic criteria.	Ann Intern Med 2005; 143:517–521 http://www.acponline.org/clinical/guidelines/?hp#general

[a]Discuss the risks, benefits, and limitations of genetic testing in patients with a positive family history of hereditary hemochromatosis or those with elevated serum ferritin level or transferrin saturation.

HEPATITIS B VIRUS INFECTION, CHRONIC

Disease Screening	Organization	Date	Population	Recommendations	Comments	Source
Hepatitis B Virus Infection, Chronic	AAFP CDC USPSTF	2007 2006 2004	Pregnant women	Screen all women with HBsAg[a] at their first prenatal visit.	USPSTF strongly recommends screening at first prenatal visit.	http://www.aafp.org/online/en/home/clinical/exam.html http://www.cdc.gov http://www.ahrq.gov/clinic/uspstf/uspshepb.htm
	AAFP USPSTF	2007 2004	General asymptomatic population	Recommends against routine screening for HBV.	Most people who become infected as adults recover fully from HBV infection and develop protective immunity.	http://www.aafp.org/online/en/home/clinical/exam.html http://www.ahrq.gov/clinic/uspstf/uspshepb.htm
	BASHH	2005	High-risk individuals[b]	Screen with HBsAg or anti-HBc.[a]	If high-risk persons are non-immune, consider vaccination.	
	CDC	2006	All infants, children, adolescents, and adults born in Asia, the Pacific Islands, Africa, and other endemic countries	Test for HBsAg.		http://www.cdc.gov/
	CDC	2006	Hemodialysis patients	Test for HBsAg.		http://www.cdc.gov/

[a]Immunoassays for HBsAg have sensitivity and specificity > 98%. (MMWR 1993;42:707)
[b]Men having sex with men; sex workers; injection drug users; HIV+ patients; sexual assault victims; people from countries where hepatitis B is common; needle-stick victims; sexual partners of high-risk persons.
BASHH = British Association for Sexual Health and HIV

HEPATITIS C VIRUS INFECTION, CHRONIC

Disease Screening	Organization	Date	Population	Recommendations	Comments	Source
Hepatitis C Virus Infection, Chronic	AAFP USPSTF	2007 2004	General population	Recommends against routine screening for HCV infection in adults who are not at increased risk.[a]	1. Seroconversion may take up to 3 months. 2. 15%–25% of persons with acute hepatitis C resolve their infection; of the remaining, 10%–20% develop cirrhosis within 20–30 years after infection, and 1%–5% develop hepatocellular carcinoma. 3. Patients testing positive for HCV antibody should receive a nucleic acid test to confirm active infection. A quantitative HCV RNA test and genotype test can provide useful prognostic information prior to initiating antiviral therapy. (JAMA 2007;297:724) 4. Also consider testing sexual partners of HCV+ persons; men having sex with men; HIV+ persons; female sex workers; tattoo recipients; alcoholics; ex-prisoners.	http://www.aafp.org/online/en/home/clinical/exam.html http://www.ahrq.gov/clinic/uspstf/uspshepc.htm
	AAFP USPSTF	2007 2004	Persons at increased risk[a]	Insufficient evidence to recommend for or against routine screening.		
	CDC	2006	Persons at increased risk[a]	Perform routine counseling, testing, and appropriate follow-up.[b] See algorithm on page 59.		http://www.cdc.gov/ncidod/diseases/hepatitis/C/plan/Prev_control.htm
	BASHH	2005	Persons at high risk[c]	Screen with antibody or HCV RNA test.		NGC Clearinghouse

[a]Increased risk includes injection drug use, receipt of clotting factor concentrates before 1987, chronic hemodialysis, receipt of blood from a donor who later tested positive for HCV, receipt of blood transfusion or organ transplant before July 1992, healthcare workers after needle sticks or mucosal exposures to HCV-positive blood, children born to HCV-positive women, and persons with evidence of chronic liver disease (abnormal ALT levels).

[b]2 types of tests are available for laboratory diagnosis of HCV infection: (1) detection of antibody to HCV antigens, and (2) detection and quantification of HCV nucleic acid. See algorithm on page 59.

[c]Injection drug users; hemophilines; blood product recipients in UK prior to 1990; needle-stick injury.

CONFIRMING HCV INFECTION IN ASYMPTOMATIC PERSONS

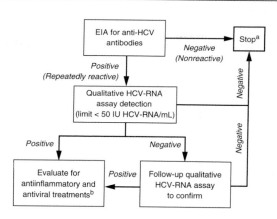

anti-HCV = antibody to HCV; EIA = enzyme immunoassay

[a]False-negative EIAs: hemodialysis or immune deficiencies.
False-positive EIAs: autoimmune disorders.

[b]Treatment recommended for those with increased risk of developing cirrhoses. Treatment with combination peg-interferon alfa-2b plus ribavirin leads to sustained virologic response in about 50% of patients with detectable HCV RNA **and** elevated ALT. (Lancet 2001;358:958) Liver biopsy is useful in demonstrating baseline abnormalities and in enabling patients and healthcare providers to decide about antiretroviral therapy. Information on viral genotype is important to guide treatment decisions.

Factors associated with successful therapy: genotypes other than 1, lower baseline viral levels, less fibrosis or inflammation on liver biopsy, lower body weight or body surface area.

Source: NIH Consens State Sci Statements. 2002 Jun 10–12;19(3):1–46; MMWR 2003;53(RR-3); Clin Liver Dis 2003;7:261.

HERPES SIMPLEX, GENITAL

Disease Screening	Organization	Date	Population	Recommendations	Comments	Source
Herpes Simplex, Genital	AAFP USPSTF	2007 2005	Adolescents and adults	Recommends against routine serological screening for HSV.	1. Seroprevalence of HSV-2 is 20% for persons > 12 years age.	http://www.aafp.org/online/home/clinical/exam.html http://www.ahrq.gov/clinic/uspstf/uspsherp.htm
	AAFP USPSTF	2007 2005	Pregnant women	Recommends against routine serological screening for HSV to prevent neonatal HSV infection.[a]	2. There is limited evidence that the use of anti-viral therapy in women with a history of recurrent HSV or performance of cesarean section in women with active HSV lesions at the the time of delivery decreases neonatal herpes infection.	

[a]Women who develop primary HSV infection during pregnancy have highest risk for transmitting HSV infection to their infants. Because these women are initially seronegative, serological screening tests do not accurately detect those at highest risk.

						HUMAN IMMUNODEFICIENCY VIRUS
Disease Screening	Organization	Date	Population	Recommendations	Comments	Source
Human Immunodeficiency Virus	AAFP USPSTF	2007 2005	Adolescents and adults at increased risk[a]	Strongly recommends screening.	1. USPSTF makes no recommendation for or against routine screening for HIV in adolescents and adults who are not at increased risk for HIV infection. 2. Initial screening test: EIA is considered reactive only when a positive result is confirmed in a second test of the original sample. Seroconversion is 95% within 6 months of infection. Specificity is > 99.5%.	http://www.aafp.org/exam/ http://www.ahrq.gov/clinic/uspstf/uspshivi.htm
	CDC	2006	Adults and adolescents (aged 13–64 years) in all healthcare settings,[c] especially persons initiating TB treatment or seeking evaluation for STD complaints	Routinely screen using "opt-out" consent.[a] Repeat screening, at least annually, of all high-risk persons.[b]	3. If acute HIV suspected, also use plasma RNA test. 4. False-positives with EIA: nonspecific reactions in persons with immunologic disturbances (eg, systemic lupus erythematosus or rheumatoid arthritis), multiple transfusions, recent influenza, or rabies vaccination. 5. Confirmatory testing is necessary using Western blot or indirect immunofluorescence assay. 6. Management of newly diagnosed HIV infection has been recently reviewed. (NEJM 2005;353: 1702–1710) 7. Awareness of HIV positivity reduces secondary HIV transmission risk and high-risk behavior and viral load if on HAART. (CDC, 2006)	MMWR 2006;55 (RR-14):1 http://www.cdc.gov/

(Comments continuation for CDC row, items overlapping): 5. risk-based testing strategies are no longer effective at reaching the majority of patients. (CDC, 2006) 6. With the evolution of HIV disease in the U.S.,

HUMAN IMMUNODEFICIENCY VIRUS

Disease Screening	Organization	Date	Population	Recommendations	Comments	Source
Human Immunodeficiency Virus (continued)	CDC	2006	All pregnant women	Include HIV testing in panel of routine prenatal screening tests. Retest high-risk women at 36 weeks' gestation.[d] Rapid HIV testing of women in labor who have not received prenatal HIV testing (opt-out screening[a]).	1. Rapid HIV antibody testing during labor identified 34 positive women among 4,849 women with no prior HIV testing documented (prevalence, 7 in 1,000). 84% of women consented to testing. Sensitivity was 100%, specificity was 99.9%, PPV was 90%. (JAMA 2004;292:219)	MMWR 2006;55 (RR-14):1
	AAFP USPSTF	2007 2005	All pregnant women	Clinicians should screen all pregnant women for HIV.		http://aafp.org/ exam/ http://www.ahrq. gov/clinic/uspstf/ uspshivi.htm

[a]HIV screening should be voluntary. Persons should be informed orally or in writing that HIV testing will be performed unless they decline (ie, opt-out screening). A separate HIV consent form is not recommended. General consent for medical care should be considered sufficient to encompass consent for HIV testing.

[b]Injection drug users and their sex partners; persons who exchange sex for money or drugs; sex partners of HIV infected persons; men having sex with men; heterosexual persons who themselves or their sex partners have had ≥ 1 sex partner since last HIV test.

[c]Unless prevalence of HIV is documented as < 0.1%.

[d]High risk includes footnote b, as well as receiving care in healthcare setting with ≥ 1 HIV case per 1,000 pregnant women per year.

EIA = enzyme immunoassay

HYPERTENSION, CHILDREN & ADOLESCENTS

Disease Screening	Organization	Date	Population	Recommendations	Comments	Source
Hypertension, Children & Adolescents	AAFP USPSTF	2007 2003	Age < 18 years	Insufficient evidence to recommend for or against routine screening for high blood pressure.	1. Hypertension: average SBP or DBP ≥ 95th percentile for gender, age, and height on ≥ 3 occasions. See Appendices. 2. Prehypertension: average SBP or DBP 90th–95th percentile. 3. Adolescents with BP ≥ 120/80 mm Hg are prehypertensive.	http://www.aafp.org/online/en/home/clinical/exam.html http://www.ahrq.gov/clinic/uspstf/uspshype.htm
	NHLBI	2004	Age 3–20 years[a]	Measure BP at least once during every health care episode.	4. Evaluation of hypertensive children: assess for additional risk factors. 5. Indications for antihypertensive drug therapy in children: symptomatic	Pediatrics 2004;114: 555–576 http://www.nhlbi.nih.gov/
	Bright Futures	2002	Age 3–21 years	Annual screening.	hypertension, secondary hypertension, target-organ damage, diabetes, persistent hypertension despite nonpharmacologic measures.	http://www.brightfutures.org

[a]In children < 3 years old, conditions that warrant BP measurement: prematurity, very low birth weight, or neonatal complications; congenital heart disease; recurrent UTI, hematuria, or proteinuria; renal disease or urologic malformations; family history of congenital renal disease; solid-organ transplant; malignancy or bone marrow transplant; drugs known to raise BP; systemic illnesses; increased intracranial pressure.

HYPERTENSION, ADULTS					
Disease Screening	Organization	Date	Population	Recommendations	Comments	Source
Hypertension, Adults	Canadian Hypertension Education Program	2007	Adults	Assess blood pressure at all appropriate clinic visits. If "high normal" (SBP 130–139, DBP 85–89), repeat annually.		http://www.hypertension.ca
	ESH ESC	2007	Adults	The diagnosis of hypertension should be based on at least 2 blood pressure measurements per visit and at least 2 to 3 visits, although in particularly severe cases the diagnosis can be based on measurements taken at a single visit.		J Hypertens 2007;25:1105 http://www.escardio.org/knowledge/guidelines/Guidelines_list.htm?hit=quick
	NICE	2006	Adults	To identify hypertension (persistent raised blood pressure above 140/90 mm Hg), ask the patient to return for at least 2 subsequent clinics where blood pressure is assessed from 2 readings under the best conditions available.		http://guidance.nice.org.uk/CG34/
	British Hypertension Society	2004	Age 18–80 years	Screen at least every 5 years. If SBP > 130 or DBP > 85, then annually.		BMJ 2004;328:634

HYPERTENSION, ADULTS

Disease Screening	Organization	Date	Population	Recommendations	Comments	Source
Hypertension, Adults (continued)	JNC VII (NHLBI)	2003	Age > 18 years	Normal: recheck in 2 years (see Comments). Prehypertension: recheck in 1 year. Stage 1 hypertension: confirm within 2 months. Stage 2 hypertension: evaluate or refer to source of care within 1 month (evaluate and treat immediately if BP > 180/110).	1. Prehypertension: SBP 120–139 or DBP 80–89. 2. Stage 1 hypertension: SBP 140–159 or DBP 90–99. 3. Stage 2 hypertension: SBP ≥ 160 or DBP ≥ 100 (based on average of ≥ 2 measurements on ≥ 2 separate office visits). 4. Perform physical exam and routine labs.[a] 5. Pursue secondary causes of hypertension.[b] 6. Treatment goals are for BP < 140/90, unless diabetes or renal disease present (< 130/80). See JNC VII Management Algorithm, page 142. 7. Ambulatory BP monitoring is a better (and independent) predictor of cardiovascular outcomes compared with office visit monitoring and is covered by Medicare when evaluating white-coat hypertension. (NEJM 2006;354:2368)	JAMA 2003;289: 2560 Hypertension 2003;42:1206
	AAFP USPSTF	2006 2003	Age ≥ 18 years	Strongly recommends screening for high blood pressure.		Hypertension 2000;35:844 NEJM 2003;348: 2407 http://www.aafp. org/online/en/ home/clinical/ exam.html http://www.ahrq. gov/clinic/uspstf/ uspshype.htm

HYPERTENSION, ADULTS

[a]Physical exam should include: measurements of height, weight, and waist circumference; funduscopic exam (retinopathy); carotid auscultation (bruit); jugular venous pulsation; thyroid gland (enlargement); cardiac auscultation (left ventricular heave, S_3 or S_4 murmurs, clicks); chest auscultation (rales, evidence of chronic obstructive pulmonary disease); abdominal exam (bruits, masses, pulsations); exam of lower extremities (diminished arterial pulsations, bruits, edema); and neurologic exam (focal findings). Routine labs include urinalysis, complete blood count, electrolytes (potassium, calcium), creatinine, glucose, fasting lipids, and 12-lead electrocardiogram.

[b]Pursue secondary causes of hypertension when evaluation is suggestive (clues in parentheses) of: (1) pheochromocytoma (labile or paroxysmal hypertension accompanied by sweats, headaches, and palpitations), (2) renovascular disease (abdominal bruits), (3) autosomal dominant polycystic kidney disease (abdominal or flank masses), (4) Cushing's syndrome (truncal obesity with purple striae), (5) primary hyperaldosteronism (hypokalemia), (6) hyperparathyroidism (hypercalcemia), (7) renal parenchymal disease (elevated serum creatinine, abnormal urinalysis), (8) poor response to drug therapy, (9) well-controlled hypertension with an abrupt increase in blood pressure, (10) SBP > 180 or DBP > 110 mm Hg, or (11) sudden onset of hypertension.

				LEAD POISONING	
Disease Screening	Organization	Date	Population	Recommendations	Comments[c]	Source
Lead Poisoning	USPSTF	2006	Childred aged 1–5 years	Insufficient evidence to recommend for or against routine screening in asymptomatic children at increased risk.[a] Recommends against screening in asymptomatic children at average risk.	1. Risk assessment should be performed during prenatal visits and continue until 6 years of age. 2. CDC personal risk questionnaire: (1) Does your child live in or regularly visit a house (or other facility, eg, daycare) that was built before 1950? (2) Does your child live in or regularly visit a house built before 1978 with recent or ongoing renovations or remodeling (within the last 6 months)? (3) Does your child have a sibling or playmate who has or did have lead poisoning? (http://www.cdc.gov/nceh/lead/guide/guide97.htm)	http://www.ahrq.gov/clinic/uspstf/uspslead.htm
	USPSTF	2006	Pregnant women	Recommends against screening in asymptomatic pregnant women.		
	AAP	2005	Infants and children	Screen Medicaid-eligible children with blood lead level at 1 and 2 years of age.[a,b] Inquire about city or state health department guidance on screening non-Medicaid-eligible children. If there is none, then consider screening all children.		Pediatrics 2005;116:1036 http://aappolicy.aappublications.org/cgi/content/full/pediatrics;116/4/1036

Disease Screening	Organization	Date	Population	Recommendations	Comments[c]	Source
LEAD POISONING						
Lead Poisoning (continued)	AAFP	2007	Infants at age 12 months	Selective screening with blood lead level for those infants at high risk. [a]		http://www.aafp.org/online/en/home/clinical/exam.html

[a]Those at increased or high risk live in communities in which the prevalence of lead levels requiring intervention is high or undefined; live in or frequently visit a home built before 1950 with dilapidated paint or with recent or ongoing renovation; have close contact with a person who has an elevated lead level; live near lead industry or heavy traffic; live with someone whose job or hobby involves lead exposure, uses lead-based pottery, or takes traditional remedies that contain lead.

[b]Confirm elevated lead levels with venous sample after screening sample from fingerstick: immediately if > 70 µg/mL, within 48 hours if 45–69 µg/mL, within 1 week if 20–44 µg/mL, and within 1 month if 10–19 µg/mL. See AAP guidelines for further treatment recommendations. See http://www.cdc.gov/nceh/lead for additional information on prevention and screening.

[c]Studies show poor rates of testing and follow-up testing in children at risk or with documented lead poisoning. (JAMA 2005;293:2232; Am J Public Health 2004;94:1945)

Disease Screening	Organization	Date	Population	Recommendations	Comments	Source
OBESITY						
Obesity	NAPNAP	2006	Children and adolescents	Calculate BMI annually being careful to ensure an accurate height and weight.	1. Additional evaluation for children and adolescents with BMI ≥ 85th percentile: focused family history for CHD risk, pulse, BP, fasting lipid profile. If risk factors, add ALT, AST, fasting glucose. If BMI > 95th percentile, add BUN, creatinine. 2. Expert Committee Classification (2007): • Obese = BMI ≥ 95th percentile for age and sex or BMI > 30. • Overweight = BMI ≥ 85th percentile but < 95th percentile for age and sex.	Extensive guidance provided in J Pediatr Health Care 2006;20 (Supplement S):1–64.
	USPSTF	2005	Children and adolescents	Insufficient evidence to recommend for or against routine screening for overweight as a means to prevent adverse health outcomes.		http://www.ahrq.gov/clinic/uspstf/uspsobch.htm
	Expert Committee on the Assessment, Prevention, and Treatment of Childhood and Adolescent Overweight and Obesity[c]	2007	Children and adolescents	Assess height, weight, BMI and plot on standard growth charts annually. Assess dietary patterns at each well-child visit. Assess physical activity at each well-child visit.		http://www.ama-assn.org/ama1/pub/upload/mm/433/ped_obesity_recs.pdf
	AAP	2003	Children and adolescents	Calculate and plot BMI annually.[a]		http://www.aap.org Pediatrics 2003;112: 424–430 NEJM 2005;352:2100–2109

Disease Screening	Organization	Date	Population	Recommendations	Comments	Source
OBESITY						
Obesity (continued)	NICE	2006	Children	Use clinical judgment to decide when to measure weight and height. • Use BMI; relate to UK 1990 BMI charts to give age- and gender-specific information. • Do not use waist circumference routinely; however, it can give information on risk of long-term health problems. • Discuss with the child and family.		http://guidance.nice.org.uk/CG43
	AAFP USPSTF	2007 2003	Age > 18 years	Recommends screening all adults and offering intensive counseling and behavioral interventions to promote sustained weight loss in obese adults.		http://www.aafp.org/online/en/home/clinical/exam.html http://www.ahrq.gov/clinic/uspstf/uspsobes.htm

Disease Screening	Organization	Date	Population	Recommendations	Comments	Source
OBESITY						
Obesity (continued)	NICE	2006	Adults	Use clinical judgment to decide when to measure weight and height. • Use BMI to classify degree of obesity but use clinical judgment. • Use waist circumference in people with a BMI <35 kg/m² to assess health risks. • Bioimpedance is not recommended as a substitute for BMI. • Tell the person his or her classification, and how this affects his or her long-term health problems.	1. See: http://www.who.int/bmi/index.jsp for the WHO Global Database on Body Mass Index. 2. See: http://www.who.int/dietphysicalactivity/en/ for the WHO statement on diet and physical activity as a public health priority. 3. BMI may be less accurate in highly muscular people. 4. For Asian adults, risk factors may be of concern at lower BMI. 5. For older people, risk factors may become important at higher BMIs.	http://guidance.nice.org.uk/CG43

Disease Screening	Organization	Date	Population	Recommendations	Comments	Source
Obesity (continued)	NHLBI	2000	Age > 18 years	Calculate BMI and measure waist circumference for all patients.[b]	1. Overweight is defined as BMI 25–29.9 kg/m^2 and obesity as BMI > 30 kg/m^2. 2. Waist–hip ratio may also provide additional prognostic information beyond BMI and waist circumference. Among women 50–69 years of age free of cancer, heart disease, and diabetes, waist–hip ratio is the best anthropometric predictor of total mortality. (Arch Intern Med 2000;160:2117) 3. Laparoscopic gastric banding was superior to orlistat/behavioral therapy, after 2 years follow-up, on the following outcomes: percent excess weight loss (87% vs. 22%), metabolic syndrome (3% vs. 24%), and quality of life. (Ann Intern Med 2006;144:625)	NHLBI. The Practical Guide: Identification, Evaluation, and Treatment of Overweight and Obesity in Adults, 2000

[a] A combination of waist circumference and BMI should be used to evaluate the presence of elevated health risk among children and adolescents. (Pediatrics 2005 Jun;115/6:1623–1630)

[b] BMI is calculated as: weight (kg)/height (m) squared. See Appendix IV for BMI Conversion Table. Studies do not support a BMI range of 25–27 as a risk factor for all-cause and cardiovascular mortality among elderly (age ≥ 65 years) persons. (Arch Intern Med 2001;161:1194) BMI cut-offs may also need to be modified for some Asian populations. (http://www.idi.org.au; Am J Clin Nutr 2001;73:123)

[c] Expert Committee participating organizations: American Academy of Child and Adolescent Psychiatry, American Academy of Pediatrics, American Association of Family Physicians, American College of Preventive Medicine, American College of Sports Medicine, American Diabetes Association, American Pediatric Surgical Association, American Psychological Association, Association of American Indian Physicians, The Endocrine Society, National Association of Pediatric Nurse Practitioners, National Association of School Nurses, National Hispanic Medical Association, National Medical Association, The Obesity Society.

OSTEOPOROSIS					
Disease Screening	Organization	Date	Population	Recommendations	Comments	Source
Osteoporosis	AAFP CTF AACE NOF USPSTF	2007 2004 2003 2003 2002	Women aged ≥ 65 years	Recommends routine[a] screening via bone mineral density (BMD).	1. The benefits of screening and treatment are of at least moderate magnitude for women at ↑ risk by virtue of age or presence of other risk factors.[b] 2. Dual energy x-ray absorptiometry (DEXA) is the most accurate clinical method for identifying those with low BMD.[c] 3. Clinical prediction rules [Simple Calculated Osteoporosis Risk Assessment Estimate (SCORE); Osteoporosis Risk Assessment Instrument (ORAI); NOF guidelines] do not perform well as a general screening method to	http://www.aafp.org/ online/en/home/clinical/ exam.html CMAJ 2004;170(11) http://www.nof.org Ann Intern Med 2002;137:526–528 http://www.aace.com/ pub/guidelines http://ahrq.gov/clinic/ uspstf/uspsoste.htm
	AAFP AACE NOF USPSTF	2006 2003 2003 2002	Women at increased risk for osteoporotic fractures[a,b,c]	Recommends routine[a] screening beginning at age 60.	identify postmenopausal women who are more likely to have osteoporosis. Are quite sensitive (98%–100%) but not specific (10–40%). (Arch Intern Med 2005;165:530–536) 4. Refer to osteoporosis screening algorithm on page 75. 5. USPSTF makes no recommendations for or against routine use of osteoporosis screening in postmenopausal women who are younger than 60 or in women 60–64 years who are not at increased risk for osteoporotic fractures.	http://www.aafp.org/ online/en/home/clinical/ exam.html http://www.nof.org Ann Intern Med 2002;137:526–528 http://www.aace.com/ pub/guidelines http://www.ahrq.gov/ clinic/uspstf/uspsoste. htm

OSTEOPOROSIS

[a] AACE recommends follow-up BMD measure in 3–5 years for women with "normal" baseline score, and if high risk, in 1–2 years.

[b] Exact risk factors that should trigger screening in this age group are difficult to specify based on evidence. Well-accepted high-risk factors include chronic steroid use (≥ 2 months), repeated fractures or fractures not caused by trauma, early menopause, blood relative with osteoporosis, known low BMD, low body weight (< 127 lb), cigarette use. See table of risk factors on page 76.

[c] Use of hip DEXA scans in > 65-year-old population associated with 36% fewer incident hip fractures over 6 years. (Am Intern Med 2005 Feb 1;142(3):173–181)

OSTEOPOROSIS: SCREENING

SELECTIVE SCREENING FOR OSTEOPOROSIS IN PERSONS NOT
CURRENTLY TAKING ANTI-OSTEOPOROSIS
MEDICATIONS OR HAVING A HISTORY OF HIP FRACTURE
[Modified from the National Osteoporosis Foundation:
Physician's guide to prevention & treatment of osteoporosis (www.nof.org); Up To Date
Screening for Osteoporosis by H.N. Rosen (www.uptodateonline.com)]

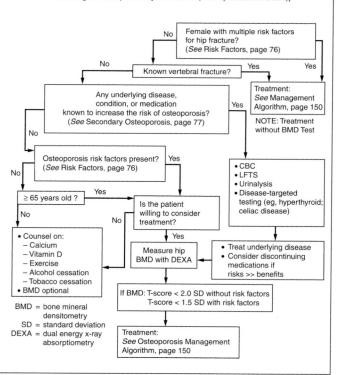

BMD = bone mineral
densitometry
SD = standard deviation
DEXA = dual energy x-ray
absorptiometry

RISK FACTORS FOR OSTEOPOROTIC FRACTURE

Potentially Modifiable	Nonmodifiable
Current cigarette smoker	*Personal history of fracture as an adult*
Low body weight (< 127 lb)	*History of fragility fracture in first-degree relative*
Oral corticosteroid use > 3 months	Caucasian race
Estrogen deficiency: -Early menopause (age < 45 years) or bilateral ovariectomy -Prolonged premenopausal amenorrhea (> 1 year)	Advanced age
	Female sex
	Dementia
Low calcium intake (lifelong)	
Alcohol (> 2 drinks/day)	
Impaired eyesight despite adequate correction	
Recurrent falls	
Inadequate physical activity	
Poor health/frailty	

Italicized items—personal or family history of fracture, smoking, and low body weight—were demonstrated in a large, ongoing, prospective U.S. study to be key factors in determining the risk of hip fracture (independent of bone density).
Source: Adapted from National Osteoporosis Foundation.
Physician's guide to prevention and treatment of osteoporosis. Available at:
http://www.nof.org/physguide, accessed July 18, 2007

CAUSES OF GENERALIZED SECONDARY OSTEOPOROSIS IN ADULTS

Drugs	Endocrine Diseases or Metabolic Causes	Collagen Vascular Diseases	Nutritional Conditions	Other Causes
Aluminum	Acromegaly	Epidermolysis bullosa	Celiac disease[a]	Amyloidosis
Anticonvulsants	Adrenal atrophy and Addison's disease	Osteogenesis imperfecta	Eating disorders	Ankylosing spondylitis
Cigarette smoking	Congenital porphyria		Gastrectomy	AIDS/HIV
Cytotoxic drugs	Cushing's syndrome		Malabsorption syndromes	Chronic obstructive pulmonary disease
Excessive alcohol	Diabetes mellitus, type 1		Nutritional disorders	Hemophilia
Excessive thyroxine	Endometriosis		Parenteral nutrition	Idiopathic scoliosis
Glucocorticosteroids & adrenocorticotropin (oral or inhaled)	Female athlete triad		Pernicious anemia	Inflammatory bowel disease
Gonadotropin-releasing hormone agonists	Gaucher's disease		Severe liver disease (especially primary biliary cirrhosis)	Lymphoma & leukemia
Heparin	Gonadal insufficiency (primary & secondary)		Sprue	Mastocytosis
Immune suppressants	Hemochromatosis			Multiple myeloma
Lithium	Hyperparathyroidism			Multiple sclerosis
Tamoxifen (premenopausal use)	Hypophosphatemia			Rheumatoid arthritis
	Thyrotoxicosis			Sarcoidosis
	Tumor secretion of parathyroid hormone–related peptide			Spinal cord transection
				Stroke
				Thalassemia

[a]Consider serologic screening of all osteoporotic patients for celiac disease. [Arch Intern Med 2005 Feb 28;165(4):393–399]
Source: Adapted from National Osteoporosis Foundation and from AACE guidelines. (Endocrin Pract 2003;9:545)
Physician's guide to prevention and treatment of osteoporosis. Available at: http://www.nof.org/physguide, accessed July 18, 2007

Disease Screening	Organization	Date	Population	Recommendations	Comments	Source
SCOLIOSIS						
Scoliosis	AAFP USPSTF	2007 2004	Asymptomatic adolescents	Recommends against routine screening for idiopathic scoliosis.	1. Positive predictive value of bending test is 42.8% for scoliosis of > 5 degrees and 6.4% for > 15 degrees; sensitivity, 74%; specificity, 78%. (Am J Public Health 1985;75:1377) 2. Recent review of scoliosis management. (J Bone Joint Surg Am 2007;89:55)	http://www.aafp.org/online/en/home/clinical/exam.html http://www.ahrq.gov/clinic/uspstf/uspsaisc.htm
	Bright Futures	2002	Adolescents	Screen during physical exam annually in adolescents and children > 8 years of age.		http://www.brightfutures.org

SPEECH & LANGUAGE DELAY

Disease Screening	Organization	Date	Population	Recommendations	Comments	Source
Speech & Language Delay	USPSTF	2006	Preschool children	Evidence is insufficient to recommend for or against routine use of brief, formal screening instruments in primary care to detect speech and language delay in children up to 5 years of age.	1. Fair evidence suggests that interventions can improve the results of short-term assessments of speech and language skills; however, no studies have assessed long-term consequences. 2. No studies have assessed any additional benefits that may be gained by treating children identified through brief, formal screening who would not be identified by addressing clinical or parental concerns. 3. No studies have addressed the potential harms of screening or interventions for speech and language delays, such as labeling, parental anxiety, or unnecessary evaluation and intervention.	http://www.ahrq. gov/clinic/uspstf/ uspschdv.htm

Disease Screening	Organization	Date	Population	Recommendations	Comments	Source
Syphilis	AAFP USPSTF	2007 2004	Pregnant women	Strongly recommends screening all pregnant women.	1. All reactive nontreponemal tests should be confirmed with a more specific treponemal test (eg, FTA-ABS). 2. Sensitivity of nontreponemal tests varies with levels of antibodies: 62%–76% in early primary syphilis, 100% during secondary syphilis, and 70% in untreated late syphilis. In late syphilis, previously reactive results revert to nonreactive in 25% of patients. 3. Specificity of nontreponemal tests is 75%–85% in persons with preexisting diseases or conditions (eg, collagen vascular diseases, injection drug use, advanced malignancy, pregnancy, malaria, tuberculosis, viral and rickettsial diseases) and 100% in persons without preexisting diseases or conditions. 4. Between 2000 and 2003, syphilis cases increased 60% in men and decreased 53% in women. About two-thirds of syphilis cases in 2003 were among men having sex with men. (Am J Public Health 2007;97:1076)	http://www.aafp.org/exam http://www.ahrq.gov/clinic/uspstf/uspssyph.htm
	AAFP USPSTF	2007 2004	Persons at increased risk[a,b]	Strongly recommends screening high-risk persons.		http://www.aafp.org/exam http://www.ahrq.gov/clinic/uspstf/uspssyph.htm
	AAN	2001	Patients with dementia	Do not screen unless clinical suspicion of neurosyphilis is present.		Neurology 2001;56:1143 http://www.aan.com/professionals/practice/guidelines/pda/Dementia_diagnosis.pdf

[a]High risk includes commercial sex workers, persons who exchange sex for money or drugs, persons with other STDs (including HIV), and sexual contacts of persons with active syphilis.
[b]Recommends against screening asymptomatic persons not at increased risk for syphilis infection.

THYROID DISEASE

Disease Screening	Organization	Date	Population	Recommendations	Comments	Source
Thyroid Disease	AAFP USPSTF	2007 2004	Adults	Insufficient evidence to recommend for or against routine screening for thyroid disease.	1. Individuals with symptoms and signs potentially attributable to thyroid dysfunction[b] and those with risk factors for its development[c] may require more frequent TSH testing. 2. When there is suspicion of pituitary or hypothalamic disease, the serum FT4 concentration should be measured in addition to the serum TSH. 3. Controversy exists regarding Rx benefit for patients with subclinical hypothyroidism (elevated TSH; normal free thyroxine). 4. RCT shows that treatment of subclinical hypothyroidism improves cardiovascular risk factors, but has small/no effect on patient-centered outcomes over 3 month period. TSH level did not predict treatment response. (J Clin Endocrinol Metab 2007;92:1715)	http://www.aafp.org/online/en/home/clinical/exam.html http://www.ahrq.gov/clinic/uspstf/uspsthyr.htm Ann Intern Med 2004;140:125–127
	ATA	2000	Women aged ≥ 35 years	Screen with serum TSH at age 35 years, and every 5 years thereafter.[a]		Arch Intern Med 2000;160:1573 http://www.thyroid.org/professionals/publications/guidelines.html
	AACE	2002	Elderly	Periodic screening with sensitive TSH.[a]		http://www.aace.com/pub/guidelines Endocr Pract 2002;8:457–469

[a] A consensus conference with representatives of ATA and AACE concluded that there is insufficient evidence to support population-based screening, but that aggressive case finding is appropriate in pregnant women, women aged > 60 years, and others at high risk for thyroid dysfunction. (JAMA 2004;291:228)

[b] Signs, symptoms, and comorbidities suggestive of hypothyroidism include previous thyroid dysfunction, goiter, surgery, or radiotherapy affecting the thyroid, diabetes mellitus, vitiligo, pernicious anemia, leukotrichia (prematurely gray hair), and medications [such as lithium carbonate and iodine-containing compounds (eg, amiodarone, radiocontrast agents, expectorants containing potassium iodide, and kelp)].

[c] Risk factors include family history of thyroid disease, or personal history of pernicious anemia, diabetes mellitus, and primary adrenal insufficiency. Laboratory test results suggestive of thyroid disease include hypercholesterolemia, hyponatremia, anemia, CPK and LDH elevations, hyperprolactinemia, hypercalcemia, alkaline phosphatase elevation, and hepatocellular enzyme elevation.

Disease Screening	Organization	Date	Population	Recommendation	Comments	Source
TOBACCO USE						
Tobacco Use	AAFP USPSTF	2007 2003	Children and adolescents	Evidence is insufficient to recommend for or against routine screening.	Teens with novelty-seeking personality traits are at increased risk of initiating and progressing in smoking behaviors. (Pediatrics 2006;117:1216)	http://www.aafp.org/online/en/home/clinical/exam.html http://www.ahrq.gov/clinic/uspstf/uspstbac.htm
	AAFP USPSTF	2007 2003	Adults	Strongly recommends screening all adults for tobacco use. See treatment advice on pages 167–168.	Smoking cessation lowers the risk of heart disease, stroke, and lung disease.	
	AAFP USPSTF	2007 2003	Pregnant women	Strongly recommends screening all pregnant women for tobacco use.	1. Extended or augmented counseling (5–15 minutes) that is tailored for pregnant smokers is more effective (17% abstinence) than generic counseling (7% abstinence). 2. Cessation during pregnancy leads to increased birth weights.	

Disease Screening	Organization	Date	Population	Recommendations	Comments	Source
Tuberculosis, Latent	AAFP ATS CDC IDSA Bright Futures	2007 2005 2005 2005 2002	Persons at increased risk of developing TB[a]	Screening by tuberculin skin test is recommended.[b,c] Frequency of testing should be based on likelihood of further exposure to TB and level of confidence in the accuracy of the results.[d]	1. Persons with (+) PPD test should receive CXR and clinical evaluation for TB. If no evidence of active infection, provide INH prophylaxis if appropriate. 2. Persons with ≥ 10 mm PPD test and who have either HIV infection or evidence of old, healed TB have the highest lifetime risk of reactivation (≥ 20%). Also at high risk (10%–20%) are those with (1) recent PPD conversion, (2) age > 35 years and immunosuppressive therapy, and (3) induration > 15 mm and age < 35 years. (NEJM 2004; 350:2060) 3. Treatment (INH for 9 months) is recommended for foreign-born persons who have latent TB infection and who have been in the United States < 5 years. 4. Prior BCG vaccination is not considered a valid basis for dismissing positive results. 5. Patients at high risk of INH liver injury should be monitored during INH therapy (history of liver disorder, HIV infection, pregnant and immediate post-partum women, regular alcohol user). [MMWR 2001;50(34)]	http://www.aafp.org/exam.xml MMWR 2005; 54(RR 12):1 http://www.thoracic.org/ http://www.cdc.gov/ http://www.brightfutures.org

[a]Increased risk: persons infected with HIV, close contacts of persons with known or suspected TB (including healthcare workers), persons with medical risk factors associated with reactivation of TB (eg, silicosis, diabetes mellitus, prolonged corticosteroid therapy, end-stage renal disease, immunosuppressive therapy), foreign-born persons from countries with high TB prevalence (eg, most countries in Africa, Asia, and Latin America), medically underserved and low-income populations, alcoholics, injection drug users, persons with abnormal CXRs compatible with past TB, and residents of long-term care facilities (eg, correctional institutions, mental institutions, nursing homes).
[b]Test: give intradermal injection of 5 U of tuberculin PPD and examine 48–72 hours later. Criteria for positive skin test (diameter of induration): > 15 mm for very high risk (HIV, abnormal CXR, recent contact with infected persons). If negative, consider 2-step testing to differentiate between booster effect and new conversion. Perform second test within 13 weeks. False-negative results occur in 5%–10%, especially early in infection, with anergy, with concurrent severe illness, in newborns and infants < 3 months old, and with improper technique.
[c]Newer serum based tests for latent TB (eg, QuantiFERON; Elisput) require further study before they can be recommended for routine screening. (Ann Intern Med 2007;146:340)
[d]Periodic (eg, at ages 1, 4–6, and 6–11 years) tuberculin skin testing is recommended for children who live in high-prevalence regions or who are otherwise at high risk.

VISUAL IMPAIRMENT, GLAUCOMA, OR CATARACT

Disease Screening	Organization	Date	Population	Recommendations	Comments	Source
Visual Impairment, Glaucoma, or Cataract	AAP	2007	Infants and children[a]	Assess for eye problems in the newborn period and then at all subsequent routine health supervision visits. Visual acuity testing beginning at age 3 years.		Ophthalmology 2003; 110:860–865 http://aappolicy. aappublications.org/cgi/ content/full/pediatrics; 111/4/902
	AAO	2007	Infants and children	Pediatric eye evaluation screening at newborn to 3 months of age, then at age 3–6 months, age 6–12 months, age 3 years, age 4 years, age 5 years, then every 1–2 years after age 5 years.		http://www.aao.org/PPP
	AOA	2002	Infants and children	Initial eye and vision screening at birth, then at age 6 months, age 3 years, and every 2 years thereafter.		http://www.aoanet.org
	AAFP USPSTF	2006 2004	Children younger than age 5 years	Recommends screening to detect amblyopia, strabismus, and defects in visual acuity.		http://www.aafp.org/ online/en/home/clinical/ exam.html http://www.ahrq.gov/ clinic/uspstf/uspsvsch. htm

VISUAL IMPAIRMENT, GLAUCOMA, OR CATARACT					
Disease Screening	Organization	Date	Population	Recommendations	Comments	Source
Visual Impairment, Glaucoma, or Cataract (continued)	AAO	2005	Adults, no risk factors	Comprehensive medical eye evaluation every 5–10 years for age < 40 years, every 2–4 years for age 40–54 years, every 1–3 years for age 55–64 years, every 1–2 years for age ≥ 65 years. [c]		http://www.aao.org/PPP
	AOA	2005	Adults, no risk factors	Comprehensive eye and vision exam every 2 years aged 18–40 years, every 2 years aged 41–60 years, and every 1 year aged ≥ 61 years. [b]		http://www.aoanet.org
	USPSTF	2005	Adults	Insufficient evidence to recommend for or against screening adults for glaucoma.		http://www.ahrq.gov/clinic/uspstf/uspsglau.htm
	AAFP	2007	Elderly	Perform routine eye and Snellen visual acuity screening.		http://www.aafp.org/online/en/home/clinical/exam.html

VISUAL IMPAIRMENT, GLAUCOMA, OR CATARACT

[a]Refer to ophthalmologist if high risk (very premature; family congenital cataracts, retinoblastoma, or metabolic or genetic diseases; significant developmental delay or neurologic difficulties; systemic disease associated with eye abnormalities).

[b]Increase frequency to every 1–2 years or as recommended for patients at risk (diabetes, hypertension, family history of ocular disease, work in occupations that are highly demanding visually or are eye hazardous, taking medications with ocular side effects, contact lens wearers, history of eye surgery, other health concerns or conditions).

[c]For patients with risk factors:

(1) Diabetes mellitus type 1: 5 years after onset then yearly.

(2) Diabetes mellitus type 2: At time of diagnosis then yearly.

(3) Diabetes mellitus before pregnancy: Before conception or early in first trimester, then every 1–12 months, dependent on extent of retinopathy.

(4) Glaucoma risk factors (elevated IOP, family history, African or Hispanic/Latino descent): Every 2–4 years for age < 40 years, every 1–3 years for age 40–54 years, every 1–2 years for age 55–64 years, every 6–12 months for age ≥ 65 years.

2
Disease Prevention

PRIMARY PREVENTION OF CANCER: NCI EVIDENCE SUMMARY (2007)

Cancer Type	Minimize Risk Factor Exposure	Strength of Evidence That Modifying or Avoiding Risk Factor Will Reduce Cancer	Therapeutic	Strength of Evidence
Breast[a,b]	Hormone replacement therapy	Solid	Tamoxifen (post-menopausal and high-risk women)	Solid
	– about 24% increased incidence of invasive breast cancer with combination HRT		Raloxifene (post-menopausal women)	Fair
			Bilateral mastectomy (high-risk women)	Solid
	Ionizing radiation	Solid	Oophorectomy (*BRCA*-positive women)	Solid
	– increased risk occurs about 10 years after exposure		Exercise	Solid
	Obesity	Uncertain	Breastfeeding	Solid
	– in WHI, RR = 2.85 for breast cancer for women > 82.2 kg compared to women < 58.7 kg			
	Alcohol	Uncertain		
	– relative risk (RR) increases about 7% for each drink per day			
Cervical	Human papillomavirus infection[c]	Solid	HPV-16/HPV-18 vaccination[d]	Fair
	Cigarette smoke	Solid	Screening with Pap smears	Solid
	High parity	Solid		
	Long-term use of oral contraceptives	Solid		
Colorectal[b,e]			*Nonsteroidal anti-inflammatory drugs*	*Inadequate[f]*
			Post-menopausal combination hormone replacement	Solid
			Polyp removal	Fair
			Low-fat, high-fiber diet	*Inadequate*

PRIMARY PREVENTION OF CANCER: NCI EVIDENCE SUMMARY (2007) (CONTINUED)				
Cancer Type	Minimize Risk Factor Exposure	Strength of Evidence That Modifying or Avoiding Risk Factor Will Reduce Cancer	Therapeutic	Strength of Evidence
Endometrial			Progesterone[g]	Solid
			Oral contraceptives	Solid
			Weight reduction	*Inadequate*
Gastric	*Helicobacter pylori* infection	Solid	*Anti-H. pylori therapy*	*Inadequate*
	Excessive salt intake	Fair	*Dietary interventions*	*Inadequate*
	Deficient consumption of fruits/vegetables	Fair		
Liver			HBV vaccination (newborns of mothers infected with HBV)	Solid
Lung	Cigarette smoking	Solid		
	Beta-carotene, pharmacological doses – in high-intensity smokers	Solid		
	Radon	Solid		
Oral	Tobacco	Solid		
	Alcohol	*Inadequate*		
Ovarian			Oral contraceptives	Solid
			Prophylactic oophorectomy – in high-risk women (eg, *BRCA-1/BRCA-2*)	Solid

PRIMARY PREVENTION OF CANCER: NCI EVIDENCE SUMMARY (2007) (CONTINUED)

Cancer Type	Minimize Risk Factor Exposure	Strength of Evidence That Modifying or Avoiding Risk Factor Will Reduce Cancer	Therapeutic	Strength of Evidence
Prostate			Finasteride (↓ incidence, but not mortality[h]) *Vitamin E* *Selenium* *Lycopene*	Solid *Inadequate* *Inadequate* *Inadequate*
Skin	*Sunburns (melanoma)*	*Inadequate*	*Sunscreen (nonmelanomatous skin cancer)*	*Inadequate*

[a]National Surgical Adjuvant Breast and Bowel Project (NSABP) Study of Tamoxifen and Raloxifene (STAR) trial: raloxifene is as effective as tamoxifen in reducing the risk of invasive breast cancer among post-menopausal women with at least a 5-year predicted breast cancer risk of 1.66% based on the Gail model. (http://bcra.nci.nih.gov/brc) Raloxifene has a lower risk of thromboembolic events and cataracts and a nonstatistically significant higher risk of noninvasive breast cancer than tamoxifen. Risk of other cancers, fractures, ischemic heart disease, and stroke is similar for both drugs. (JAMA 2006;295:2727) The National Cancer Institute is supporting a number of ongoing breast cancer prevention trials. (http://www.cancer.gov/clinicaltrials)

[b]Women's Health Initiative (WHI): alternate-day use of low-dose aspirin (100 mg) for an average of 10 years of treatment does not lower risk of total, breast, colorectal, or other site-specific cancers. There was a trend toward reduction in risk for lung cancer. (JAMA 2005;294:47–55)

[c]Methods to minimize risk of HPV infection include abstinence from sexual activity and the use of barrier contraceptives and/or spermicidal gel during sexual intercourse.

[d]On June 8, 2006, the U.S. Food and Drug Administration (FDA) announced approval of Gardasil, the first vaccine developed to prevent cervical cancer, precancerous genital lesions, and genital warts due to human papillomavirus (HPV) types 6, 11, 16, and 18. The vaccine is approved for use in females 9–26 years of age. (http://www.fda.gov) GlaxoSmithKline is testing a bivalent vaccine against HPV types 16 and 18. (NEJM 2006;354:1109–1112)

[e]Cereal fiber supplementation and diets low in fat and high in fiber, fruits, and vegetables do not reduce the rate of adenoma recurrence over a 3-year to 4-year period.

[f]There is solid evidence that NSAIDs reduce the risk of adenomas, but the extent to which this translates into a reduction in colorectal cancer is uncertain.

[g]Progesterone eliminates risk of endometrial cancer associated with unopposed estrogen use.

[h]Finasteride treatment increased erectile dysfunction, loss of libido, and gynecomastia.

Source: http://www.cancer.gov/cancertopics/pdq/prevention.

DIABETES, TYPE 2					

Disease Prevention	Organization	Date	Population	Recommendations	Comments	Source
Diabetes, Type 2	ADA	2007	Patients with impaired fasting glucose or glucose tolerance (see page 47)	Counsel on increasing physical activity and weight loss. Follow-up counseling important for success. Monitor for diabetes every 1–2 years. Pay close attention to, and treat, other CVD risk factors (eg, tobacco use, hypertension, dyslipidemia).	1. Drug therapy should not be routinely used to prevent diabetes until more information is known about cost-effectiveness. 2. RCTs have proven the efficacy of increased physical activity (at least 30 minutes daily) and weight loss (at least 5%–10% body weight) for preventing type 2 diabetes. Maintenance of modest weight loss through diet and physical activity reduces incidence of type 2 DM in high-risk persons by 40%–60% over 3–4 years. (Ann Intern Med 2004;140: 951)	Diabetes Care 2007;30 (Suppl 1) http://www.diabetes.org/for-health-professionals-and-scientists/cpr.jsp

ENDOCARDITIS

Disease Prevention	Organization	Date	Population	Recommendations	Comments	Source
Endocarditis	AHA	2007	Persons at highest risk for adverse events[a]	Give antibiotic prophylaxis[b] before certain dental[c] as well as certain other procedures.[d]	Major departure from previous guidelines is emphasis on providing prophylaxis to patients at greatest risk of complications of endocarditis, rather than at greatest lifetime risk of endocarditis.	Circulation 2007;115, e-published April 19, 2007

[a]Patients with prosthetic valve; previous endocarditis; selected patients with congenital heart disease (unrepaired cyanotic CHD; completely repaired congenital heart defect with prosthetic material or device during first 6 months after procedure; repaired cyanotic CHD with residual defects at or near repair site); and cardiac transplant recipients who develop valvulopathy.

[b]Standard prophylaxis regimen: amoxicillin (adults 2.0 g; children 50 mg/kg orally 1 hour before procedure). If unable to take oral medications, give ampicillin (adults 2.0 g IM or IV; children 50 mg/kg IM or IV within 30 minutes of procedure). If penicillin-allergic, give clindamycin (adults 600 mg; children 20 mg/kg orally 1 hour before procedure) or azithromycin or clarithromycin (adults 500 mg; children 15 mg/kg orally 1 hour before procedure). If penicillin-allergic and unable to take oral medications, give clindamycin (adults 600 mg; children 20 mg/kg IV within 30 minutes before procedure). If allergy to penicillin is not anaphylaxis, angioedema, or urticaria, options for non-oral treatment also include cefazolin (1 g IM or IV for adults, 50 mg/kg IM or IV for children); and for penicillin-allergic oral therapy includes cephalexin 2 g PO for adults or 50 mg/kg PO for children.

[c]All dental procedures that involve manipulation of gingival tissue or the periapical region of teeth or perforation of oral mucosa.

[d]Antibiotic prophylaxis may be reasonable for procedures in the respiratory tract or infected skin, skin structures, or musculoskeletal tissue. Antibiotic prophylaxis solely to prevent endocarditis is *not* recommended for GU or GI procedures.

FALLS IN THE ELDERLY

Older person who:
- Presents for medical attention due to a fall, or
- Reports ≥ 1 fall in past year, or
- Demonstrates abnormalities of gait and/or balance

↓

Fall evaluation:
- History: fall circumstances, medications, acute or chronic medical problems, mobility
- Exam: vision, gait and balance, lower extremity joint function, neurologic function (mental status; muscle strength; lower extremity peripheral nerves; proprioception; reflexes; cortical, extrapyramidal, and cerebellar function), cardiovascular status (heart rate and rhythm, postural pulse and blood pressure, heart rate and blood pressure response to carotid sinus stimulation)

↓

Multifactorial interventions:
(as appropriate, based on evaluation)
- Appropriate use of assistive devices
- Exercise programs, with balance training
- Gait training
- Modification of environmental hazards
- Review and modification of medications, especially psychotropics
- Staff education at long-term care and assisted-living settings
- Treatment of cardiovascular disorders
- Treatment of postural hypotension

Source: JAGS 2001;49:664–672 and NEJM 2003;348:42–49.

HYPERTENSION						
Disease Prevention	Organization	Date	Population	Recommendations	Comments	Source
Hypertension	Canadian Hypertension Education Program JNC VII NHLBI	2007 2003 2003	Persons at risk for developing hypertension[a]	Recommend weight loss, reduced sodium intake, moderate alcohol consumption, increased physical activity, potassium supplementation, modification of eating patterns.[b]	1. A 5 mm Hg reduction of SBP in the population would result in a 14% overall reduction in mortality due to stroke, a 9% reduction in mortality due to coronary heart disease, and a 7% decrease in all-cause mortality. 2. Weight loss of as little as 10 lb (4.5 kg) reduces BP and/or prevents hypertension in a large proportion of overweight patients.	http://www. hypertension.ca Hypertension 2003;42: 1206–1252

[a]Family history of hypertension; African-American (black race) ancestry; overweight or obesity; sedentary lifestyle; excess intake of dietary sodium; insufficient intake of fruits, vegetables, and potassium; excess consumption of alcohol.
[b]See Lifestyle Modifications for Primary Prevention of Hypertension on page 95.

LIFESTYLE MODIFICATIONS FOR PRIMARY PREVENTION OF HYPERTENSION

- Maintain normal body weight for adults (BMI, 18.5–24.9 kg/m^2)

- Reduce dietary sodium intake to no more than 100 mmol/day (approximately 6 g of sodium chloride or 2.4 g of sodium/day)

- Engage in regular aerobic physical activity such as brisk walking (at least 30 minutes/day, most days of the week)

- Limit alcohol consumption to no more than 2 drinks [eg, 24 oz (720 mL) of beer, 10 oz (300 mL) of wine, or 3 oz (90 mL) of 100-proof whiskey] per day in most men and to no more than 1 drink per day in women and lighter-weight persons

- Maintain adequate intake of dietary potassium [> 90 mmol (3,500 mg)/day]

- Consume a diet that is rich in fruits and vegetables and in low-fat dairy products with a reduced content of saturated and total fat [Dietary Approaches to Stop Hypertension (DASH) eating plan]

- Maintain a smoke-free environment

Source: http://www.hypertension.ca
Hypertension 2003;42:1206–1252
Trials of Hypertension Prevention (TDHP) long-term follow-up: risk of cardiovascular event 25% lower in sodium reduction group (relative risk, 0.75; 95% CI, 0.57–0.99) (BMJ 2007;334:885–892)

					MYOCARDIAL INFARCTION	

Disease Prevention	Organization	Date	Population	Recommendations	Comments	Source
Myocardial Infarction	*In a recent report showing a 50% reduction in the population's CHD mortality, 81% was attributable to primary prevention of CHD through tobacco cessation and lipid- and blood pressure–lowering activities. Only 19% of CHD mortality reduction occurred in patients with existing CHD (secondary prevention).*					BMJ 2005;331 (7517):614
	USPSTF	2002	Adults at increased risk of CHD events	Strongly recommends consideration of aspirin chemoprevention; optimum dose is unknown.	1. Meta-analysis concludes aspirin prophylaxis reduces ischemic stroke risk in women (−17%) and MI events in men (−32%). No mortality benefit in either group. Risk of bleeding increased in both groups to a similar degree as the event rate reduction. (JAMA 2006;295:306–313) 2. New tests being developed to identify high-risk individuals: noninvasive testing for skin tissue cholesterol; inflammatory markers (high-sensitivity C-reactive protein, interleukin-6, serum amyloid A), multislice computed tomography, leukocyte subtypes. [JAMA 2005; 293:2582–2583; JAMA 2005;293 (20):2471–2478; J Am Coll Cardiol 2005;45(10):1638–1643]	http://www.ahrq.gov/clinic/uspstf/uspsasmi.htm
	AHA	2006	All children and adults	*Dietary guidelines*: (1) Balance calorie intake and physical activity to achieve or maintain a healthy body weight. (2) Consume a diet rich in vegetables and fruit. (3) Choose whole grain, high-fiber foods. (4) Consume fish, especially oily fish, at least twice a week. (5) Limit intake of saturated fat to < 7% energy, trans fat to < 1% energy, and cholesterol to < 300 mg per day by • choosing lean meats and vegetable alternatives • selecting fat free (skim), 1% fat, and low-fat dairy products • minimizing intake of partially hydrogenated fats		Circulation 2002;106:388 Circulation 2006;114:82–96 http://www.americanheart.org

				MYOCARDIAL INFARCTION		

Disease Prevention	Organization	Date	Population	Recommendations	Comments	Source
Myocardial Infarction (continued)	AHA (continued)			(6) Minimize intake of beverages and foods with added sugars. (7) Choose and prepare foods with little or no salt. (8) If you consume alcohol, do so in moderation. (9) Follow these recommendations for food consumed/prepared inside *and* outside of the the home. *Avoid use of and exposure to tobacco products.*		
	AHA NCEP III	2002 2002	Hyperlipidemia[a]	For screening recommendations, see page 38; also see NCEP III screening and management (page 127) recommendations.	1. Short-term reduction in LDL using dietary counseling by dietitians is superior to that achieved by physicians. (Am J Med 2000;109:549) 2. PROVE IT–TIMI22: Lowest rate of recurrent events (1.9/100 person-years) when LDL < 70 mg/dL and CRP < 1 mg/L after statin therapy. [NEJM 2005;352(1):20–28]	Circulation 2002; 106:338 Circulation 2004; 110:227–239

MYOCARDIAL INFARCTION						
Disease Prevention	**Organization**	**Date**	**Population**	**Recommendations**	**Comments**	**Source**
Myocardial Infarction (continued)	JNC VII	2003	Hypertension	See page 142 for JNC VII treatment algorithms.	1. Antiplatelet therapy with ASA not recommended for primary prevention of MI in hypertensive patients (benefit negated by harm). Antiplatelet therapy recommended for secondary prevention. Glycoprotein IIb/IIIa inhibitors, ticlopidine, and clopidogrel have not been sufficiently evaluated in patients with hypertension. (Cochrane Database Syst Rev 2004;3:CD003186) 2. If SBP ≥ 160 mm Hg or DBP ≥ 100 mm Hg, then start with 2 drugs.	Hypertension 2003;42:1206–1252
	AHA	2007	Hypertension	Goal: < 140/90 for general population; < 130/80 if high CHD risk [diabetes, chronic kidney CHD or CHD equivalent (carotid artery disease, peripheral arterial disease, abdominal aortic aneurysm), or 10-year Framingham risk score $\geq 10\%$]. (See Appendix)		Circulation 2007; 115:2761–2788

MYOCARDIAL INFARCTION

Disease Prevention	Organization	Date	Population	Recommendations	Comments	Source
Myocardial Infarction (continued)	ACP	2004	Diabetes	Statins should be used for primary prevention of macrovascular complications if patient has type 2 DM and other cardiovascular risk factors (age > 55 years, left ventricular hypertrophy, previous cerebrovascular disease, peripheral arterial disease, smoking, or hypertension).		Ann Intern Med 2004;140:644–649 http://www.acponline.org/clinical/guidelines/?hp#acg
	ADA AHA	2007 2006	Diabetes	Goals: normal fasting glucose ($\leq$ 100 mg/dL) and near normal HbA$_{1c}$ (< 7%), BP < 130/80 mm Hg; LDL–C < 100 mg/dL (or < 70 for high risk). Aspirin therapy (75–162 mg/day) for those at increased risk. Advise all patients not to smoke.	1. Diabetes with BP 130–139/80–89 that persists after 3 months of lifestyle and behavioral therapy should be treated with agents that block the renin-angiotensin system. If BP > 140/90, treat with drug class demonstrated to reduce CHD events in diabetics (ACE inhibitors, angiotensin receptor blockers, beta-blockers, diuretics, and calcium channel blockers). 2. Improved outcomes demonstrated for lower BP targets (< 130/80 mm Hg). [Diabetes Care 2002;25(Suppl 1):S71]	Diabetes Care 2007;30:Suppl1 Circulation 2006;114:82–96 http://www.americanheart.org

| | | | | MYOCARDIAL INFARCTION | | |

Disease Prevention	Organization	Date	Population	Recommendations	Comments	Source
Myocardial Infarction (continued)	AHA	2007	Women	In addition to standard recommendations, highlight: Waist circumference ≤ 35 in. Omega-3 fatty acids if high risk.[a] BP < 120/80. Lipids: LDL-C < 100 mg/dL, HDL-C > 50 mg/dL, triglycerides < 150 mg/dL. Aspirin (75–325 mg); or clopidogrel if high-risk[a] woman is intolerant of aspirin (not recommended if low risk). ACE inhibitors if high risk.[a] Depression referral/treatment. Estrogen plus progestin hormone therapy should NOT be used or continued. Antioxidants, folic acid, and B_{12} supplementation are NOT recommended to prevent CHD.	In women ≥ 65 years, *consider* aspirin (81 mg daily or 100 mg every other day) if blood pressure is controlled and benefit for ischemic stroke and MI prevention is likely to outweigh risk of GI bleed and hemorrhagic stroke.	Circulation 2007;115:1481–1501 http://www.americanheart.org

[a]High risk: CHD or risk equivalent or 10-year absolute CHD risk > 20%.

OSTEOPOROTIC HIP FRACTURE

Disease Prevention	Organization	Date	Population	Recommendations	Comments	Source
Osteoporotic Hip Fracture	AAFP AACE NOF NIH	2007 2003 2003 2001	All women	Counsel all women about fracture risk reduction (dietary calcium, vitamin D, weight-bearing exercise, smoking cessation, moderate alcohol intake, fall risk reduction).[a,b]	1. See page 77 for medical disorders associated with osteoporosis. 2. For women receiving thyroid replacement therapy for nonmalignant conditions, periodically monitor TSH levels and adjust dose. 3. Statin use did not improve fracture risk or bone density in the Women's Health Initiative Observational Study. (Ann Intern Med 2003;139:97–104)	http://www.aafp.org/online/en/home/clinical/exam.html http://www.nof.org/ JAMA 2001;285:785–795 Endocrine Practice 2003;9(6):545–564 NEJM 2001;345:941–947; 989–992 http://www.aace.com/pub/guidelines
	NICE	2007	Women[e] with T-score < −2.55	Treatment with alendronate is recommended as first-line therapy for the following group of women: ≥ 70 years if ≥ 1 fracture risk factor[c] or ≥ 1 low BMD risk factor.[d] < 70 years post-menopausal if ≥ 1 fracture risk factor[c] and ≥ 1 low BMD risk factor.		http://guidance.nice.org.uk/page.aspx?o=437520
	CTF	2004	Women with T-score < −2.55	Treat with alendronate, risedronate, or raloxifene[f]; repeat DEXA in 1–2 years.		CMAJ 2004;170:1665

					OSTEOPOROTIC HIP FRACTURE	

Disease Prevention	Organization	Date	Population	Recommendations	Comments	Source
Osteoporotic Hip Fracture (continued)	AACE	2003		See Management algorithm page 150.		

[a]Recommended calcium: 9–18 years, 1,500 mg/day; 19–50 years, 1,000 mg/day; > 50 years, 1,200 mg/day. Recommended vitamin D: 400–800 IU/day. Use of alcohol and caffeine-containing beverages is inconsistently associated with decreased bone mass. Grip strength and current exercise are associated with increased bone mass.

[b]Calcium from dietary sources appears to result in greater BMD than calcium through supplementation. (Am J Clin Nutr 2007;85:1428)

[c](NICE) Hip fracture risk factors include parental history of hip fracture, alcohol intake ≥ 4 units/day, and severe/long-term rheumatoid arthritis.

[d](NICE) Low BMD risk factors include BMI < 22 kg/m^2, medical conditions that result in prolonged immobility, and untreated premature menopause.

[e]Does not apply to women with prior osteoporotic fracture, or women taking chronic corticosteriod therapy, and assumes women are calcium and vitamin D replete.

[f]Second-line agents include etidronate, oral pamidronate, and PTH; last-line agents are HRT or calcitonin.

OSTEOPOROTIC HIP FRACTURE: PREVENTION FOR WOMEN AT RISK*

1. <u>COUNSEL ON:</u>
   - Tobacco cessation
   - Limit alcohol intake
   - Regular weight-bearing exercise ≥ 30 min. 3x/week
   - Muscle strengthening exercise
   - Adequate Ca^{2+} intake 1,000–1,200 mg/day
   - Adequate vitamin D 800 IU/day

2. <u>IDENTIFY AND REMEDY</u>
   <u>SECONDARY CAUSES</u>
   (see table, page 77)

PERIMENOPAUSAL/POST-MENOPAUSAL	ELDERLY

PERIMENOPAUSAL/POST-MENOPAUSAL
- Identify and treat sensory deficits, neurologic disease & arthritis, all of which can lead to ↑ frequency of falls
- Adjust drug dosages for drugs that are sedating, slow reflexes, ↓ coordination & impair a person's ability to break impact of a fall
- Gait & balance training to ↓ risk of falls
- Identify and treat ♀ with osteoporosis-related fractures and those with low bone mass.

ELDERLY
- See perimenopausal/postmenopausal recommendations; in addition:
- Anchor rugs
- Minimize clutter
- Remove loose wires
- Use non-skid mats
- Add handrails in halls, bathrooms, & stairwells
- Ensure adequate lighting in halls, stairwells, & entrances
- Wear sturdy, low-heeled shoes

Source: Adapted from AACE clinical practice guidelines for the prevention & treatment of postmenopausal osteoporosis. [Endocrine Practice 2003;9(6):545–564]

*See page 76 for description of risks.

					STROKE	
Disease Prevention	Organization	Date	Population	Recommendations	Comments	Source
Stroke[a]	AHA/ASA	2006	Hypertension	Screen and treat in accordance with JNC VII (pages 142–144).		http://www.americanheart.org Stroke 2006;37:1583–1633
	ACP	2003	Atrial fibrillation	Prioritize rate control; de-emphasize rhythm.	1. Average stroke rate in patients with risk factors about 5% per year. 2. Meta-analysis: Adjusted-dose warfarin and antiplatelet agents reduce absolute	http://www.acponline.org/clinical/guidelines/?hp#acg Ann Intern Med 2003;139:1009
	ACCP	2004	Atrial fibrillation	Give anticoagulation with warfarin; target prothrombin time INR = 2.5 (range, 2.0–3.0) as noted below: All patients with any high-risk factor for stroke[b] or > 1 moderate risk factor for stroke[c]: Give warfarin as above. Patients with 1 moderate risk factor[c]: Give aspirin or warfarin as above. Patients with no high or moderate risk factors: Give aspirin, 325 mg/day.	risk of stroke [adjusted dose warfarin vs. placebo or no treatment, absolute risk reduction = 2.7% per year (NNT = 37); antiplatelet agents vs. placebo or no treatment, absolute risk reduction = 0.8% per year (NNT = 125); adjusted-dose	Chest 2004;126:429S–456S
	ACC/AHA/ESC	2006	Atrial fibrillation	1. Antithrombotic therapy recommended for all patients with atrial fibrillation, except those with lone atrial fibrillation or contraindications. 2. See Management algorithm, page 117, for medication and dosing recommendations.	warfarin vs. antiplatelet therapy, absolute risk reduction = 0.9% per year (NNT = 111)]. Risk of intracranial hemorrhage or major extracranial hemorrhage = 0.2%–0.3% per year (NNH = 333–500). (Ann Intern Med 2007;146:857–867)	Stroke 2006;37:1583–1633 Circulation 2006;114:e257–e354

STROKE					
Disease Prevention[a]	**Organization**	**Date**	**Population**	**Recommendations**	**Comments**	**Source**
Stroke[a] **(continued)**	AHA/ASA	2006	Diabetes	1. Endorse tight control of BP per JNC VII. 2. Statin therapy. 3. Consider ACE inhibitor or ARB therapy for further stroke risk reduction.		http://www.myamericanheart.org/portal/professional/guidelines Stroke 2006;37:1583–1633
	AHA/ASA	2006	Asymptomatic carotid artery stenosis	1. Screen asymptomatic CAS for other stroke risk factors and treat aggressively. 2. Aspirin unless contraindicated. 3. Prophylactic CEA for patients with high-grade (> 60%) CAS when performed by surgeons with low (< 3%) morbidity/mortality rates.	Clear consensus exists on efficacy of treatment for symptomatic CAS; treatment of asymptomatic CAS is controversial.[d] Atherosclerotic intracranial stenosis: Aspirin (1,300 mg/day) should be used in preference to warfarin. Warfarin—significantly higher rates of adverse events with no benefit over aspirin. [NEJM 2005 Mar 31;352(13):1305–1316]	http://www.myamericanheart.org/portal/professional/guidelines Stroke 2006;37:1583–1633

Disease Prevention[a]	Organization	Date	Population	Recommendations	Comments	Source
STROKE						
Stroke[a] (continued)	AHA/ASA	2006	Hyperlipidemia	See screening recommendations on page 38. See Cholesterol and Lipid Management (pages 127–129). Statin initiation per NCEP III for high stroke risk hypertensive patients with upper limit LDL is recommended.		Stroke 2006;37: 1583–1633
	AHA/ASA	2006	Sickle cell disease	Begin screening with transcranial Doppler (TCD) at 2 years of age. Transfusion therapy is recommended for patients at high stroke risk per TCD (high cerebral blood flow velocity > 200 cm/second). Frequency of screening not determined.	Transfusion therapy decreased stroke rates from 10% to < 1% per year. (NEJM 1998;339:5)	Stroke 2006;37: 1583–1633
	AHA/ASA	2006	Smoking	Strongly encourage patient and family to stop smoking. Provide counseling, nicotine replacement, and formal programs as available. Avoid environmental smoke.		Stroke 2006;37: 1583–1633

[a]Assess risk of stroke in all patients. See Appendix VI for risk assessment tool.
[b]High-risk factors for stroke in patients with atrial fibrillation include previous transient ischemic attack or stroke or embolus, hypertension, poor LV function, age > 75 years, diabetes, rheumatic mitral valve disease, and prosthetic heart valves.
[c]Moderate risk factors for stroke are age 65–75 years, diabetes, and coronary artery disease with preserved LV function.
[d]Net benefit of carotid endarterectomy requires treatment by surgical team with low perioperative risk of stroke/death (< 3%) and is enhanced for patients with symptomatic CAS when performed early (within 2 weeks of last ischemic event). (Lancet 2004;363:915) CEA remains the standard of care, even in high-risk surgical patients. [Ann Surg 2005 Feb;241(2):356–363]

3
Disease Management

ALCOHOL DEPENDENCE: EVALUATION & MANAGEMENT
Source: NIAAA, 2005

How to Screen for Heavy Drinking
Step 1: Ask About Alcohol Use

Ask: Do you sometimes drink beer, wine or other alcoholic beverages?

(No)   (Yes)

Screening complete

Ask the screening question about heavy drinking days:
How many times in the past year have you had...

5 or more	**4 or more**
drinks in a day?	drinks in a day?
(for men)	*(for women)*

One standard drink is equivalent to 12 ounces of beer, 5 ounces of wine, or 1.5 ounces of 80-proof spirits.

Is the answer 1 or more times?

(No)   (Yes)

- Advise staying within maximum drinking limits:

  For healthy men up to age 65—
  - no more than 4 drinks in a day AND
  - no more than 14 drinks in a week

  For healthy women (and healthy men over age 65)—
  - no more than 3 drinks in a day AND
  - no more than 7 drinks in a week

- Recommend lower limits or abstinence as indicated; for example, for patients who take medications that interact with alcohol, have a health condition exacerbated by alcohol, or are pregnant (advise abstinence)

- Rescreen annually

- Your patient is an at-risk drinker. For a more complete picture of the drinking pattern, determine the weekly average:

  - On average, how many days a week do you have an alcoholic drink? ☐

  - On a typical drinking day, how many drinks do you have? ☐

    Weekly average: ☐

- Record heavy drinking days in past year and weekly average in chart.

Go to Step 2

ALCOHOL DEPENDENCE: EVALUATION & MANAGEMENT (CONTINUED)
Source: NIAAA, 2005

Step 2: Assess for Alcohol Use Disorders

Next, determine if there is a maladaptive pattern of alcohol use, causing clinically significant impairment or distress.

Determine whether, in the past 12 months, your patient's drinking has repeatedly caused or contributed to

- ☐ risk of bodily harm (drinking and driving, operating machinery, swimming)
- ☐ relationship trouble (family or friends)
- ☐ role failure (interference with home, work, or school obligations)
- ☐ run-ins with the law (arrests or other legal problems)

If yes to one or more → your patient has **alcohol abuse**.

In either case, proceed to assess for dependence symptoms.

Determine whether, in the past 12 months, your patient has

- ☐ not been able to stick to drinking limits (repeatedly gone over them)
- ☐ not been able to cut down or stop (repeated failed attempts)
- ☐ shown tolerance (needed to drink a lot more to get the same effect)
- ☐ shown signs of withdrawal (tremors, sweating, nausea, or insomnia when trying to quit or cut down)
- ☐ kept drinking despite problems (recurrent physical or psychological problems)
- ☐ spent a lot of time drinking (or anticipating or recovering from drinking)
- ☐ spent less time on other matters (activities that had been important or pleasurable)

If yes to three or more → your patient has **alcohol dependence**.

Does patient meet criteria for abuse or dependence?

(No)

(Yes)

**Go to page 110
for at-risk drinking**

**Go to page 111
for alcohol use disorders**

ALCOHOL DEPENDENCE: EVALUATION & MANAGEMENT (CONTINUED)
Source: NIAAA, 2005

For At-Risk Drinking (no abuse or dependence)
Step 3: Advise and Assist

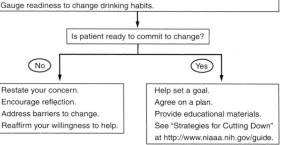

State your conclusion and recommendation clearly and relate them to patient concerns or medical findings.
Gauge readiness to change drinking habits.

Is patient ready to commit to change?

No

Yes

Restate your concern.
Encourage reflection.
Address barriers to change.
Reaffirm your willingness to help.

Help set a goal.
Agree on a plan.
Provide educational materials.
See "Strategies for Cutting Down" at http://www.niaaa.nih.gov/guide.

Step 4: At Follow-Up: Continue Support

Reminder: Document alcohol use and review goals at each visit.

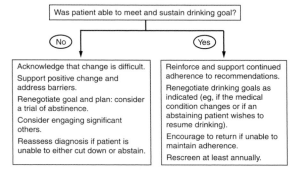

Was patient able to meet and sustain drinking goal?

No

Yes

Acknowledge that change is difficult.
Support positive change and address barriers.
Renegotiate goal and plan: consider a trial of abstinence.
Consider engaging significant others.
Reassess diagnosis if patient is unable to either cut down or abstain.

Reinforce and support continued adherence to recommendations.
Renegotiate drinking goals as indicated (eg, if the medical condition changes or if an abstaining patient wishes to resume drinking).
Encourage to return if unable to maintain adherence.
Rescreen at least annually.

ALCOHOL DEPENDENCE: EVALUATION & MANAGEMENT (CONTINUED)
Source: NIAAA, 2005

For Alcohol Use Disorders (abuse or dependence)
Step 3: Advise and Assist

- State your conclusion and recommendation clearly and relate them to medical concerns or findings.
- Negotiate a drinking goal.
- Consider evaluation by an addiction specialist.
- Consider recommending a mutual help group. For patients who have dependence, consider:
  - the need for medially managed withdrawal (detoxification) and treat accordingly.
  - prescribing a medication for alcohol dependence for patients who endorse abstinence as a goal. See page 112.
- Arrange follow-up appointments.

Step 4: At Follow-Up: Continue Support

Reminder: Document alcohol use and review goals at each visit.

> Was patient able to meet and sustain drinking goal?

(No) (Yes)

No	Yes
Acknowledge that change is difficult.	Reinforce and support continued adherence.
Support efforts to cut down or abstain.	Coordinate care with specialists as appropriate.
Relate drinking to ongoing problems as appropriate.	Maintain medications for alcohol dependence for at least 3 months and as clinically indicated thereafter.
Consider (if not yet done): consulting with an addiction specialist. recommending a mutual help group engaging significant others. prescribing a medication for alcohol dependence for patients who endorse abstinence as a goal.	Treat coexisting nicotine dependence.
Address coexisting disorders as needed.	Address coexisting disorders as needed.

PRESCRIBING MEDICATIONS

The chart below contains excerpts from page 16 of NIAAA's *Helping Patients Who Drink Too Much: A Clinical Guide* (http://www.niaaa.nih.gov/guide). It does not provide complete information and is not meant to be a substitute for the patient package inserts or other drug references used by clinicians. Behavioral support recommended.

	Disulfiram (Antabuse®)	Naltrexone (ReVia®, Depade®) and Extended-Release Injectable Naltrexone (Vivitrol®)	Acamprosate (Campral®)
Contraindications	Concomitant use of alcohol or alcohol-containing preparations or metronidazole; coronary artery disease; severe myocardial disease; hypersensitivity to rubber (thiuram) derivatives	Currently using opioids or in acute opioid withdrawal; anticipated need for opioid analgesics; acute hepatitis or liver failure	Severe renal impairment (CrCl ≤ 30 mL/min)
Key precautions	Psychoses (current or history); hepatic dysfunction; cerebral damage; diabetes; epilepsy; hypothyroidism; renal impairment; pregnancy category C	Other hepatic disease; renal impairment; history of suicide attempts or depression; pregnancy category C. If opioid analgesia is required, larger doses may be required, and respiratory depression may be deeper and more prolonged.	Moderate renal impairment (dose adjustment for CrCl 30–50 mL/min); depression or suicidality; pregnancy category C
More common serious adverse reactions	Disulfiram-alcohol reaction; hepatitis; peripheral neuropathy; psychotic reactions; optic neuritis	Will precipitate severe withdrawal if patient is dependent on opioids; hepatotoxicity (uncommon at usual doses)	Rare suicidal ideation and behavior
Common side effects	Metallic after-taste; dermatitis; drowsiness	*Nausea*; vomiting; dizziness; headache; anxiety and fatigue	*Diarrhea*; somnolence
Examples of drug interactions	Warfarin; isoniazid; metronidazole; any nonprescription drug containing alcohol; phenytoin	Opioid analgesics (blocks action)	No clinically relevant interactions known

PRESCRIBING MEDICATIONS (CONTINUED)			
	Disulfiram (Antabuse®)	**Naltrexone (ReVia®, Depade®) and Extended-Release Injectable Naltrexone (Vivitrol®)**	**Acamprosate (Campral®)**
How to prescribe	*Oral dose*: 250 mg daily (range, 125 mg to 500 mg)	*Oral dose*: 50 mg daily *IM dose*: 380 mg as deep intramuscular injection, once monthly	*Oral dose*: 666 mg (two 333-mg tablets) three times daily or, for patients with moderate renal impairment (CrCl 30–50 mL/min), reduce to 333 mg (one tablet) three times daily
	Before prescribing: (1) Warn that patient should not take disulfiram for at least 12 hours after drinking and that a disulfiram-alcohol reaction can occur up to 2 weeks after the last dose; and (2) warn about alcohol in the diet (eg, sauces and vinegars) and in medications and toiletries	*Before prescribing*: Evaluate for possible current opioid use; consider a urine toxicology screen for opioids, including synthetic opioids. Obtain liver function tests.	*Before prescribing*: Establish abstinence
	Follow-up: Monitor liver function tests periodically. Advise patient to carry a wallet card.	*Follow-up*: Monitor liver function tests periodically. Advise patient to carry a wallet card.	

Note: Whether or not a medication should be prescribed and in what amount is a matter between individuals and their healthcare providers. The prescribing information provided here is not a substitute for a provider's judgment in an individual circumstance, and the NIH accepts no liability or responsibility for use of the information with regard to particular patients.

ASTHMA MANAGEMENT ALGORITHM FOR ADOLESCENTS AND ADULTS (AGE ≥ 12 YEARS)
Source: NHLBI, 2007

Assess asthma control

	Well controlled	Not well controlled	Poorly controlled
Symptoms per week	≤ 2 days	> 2 days	every day
Nighttime awakening	≤ 2/month	1–3/week	≥ 4/week
Activity interference	none	some	a lot
prn SABA use	≤ 2 days/week	> 2 days/week	every day
FEV-1 or peak flow	> 80%	60–80%	< 60%
Oral steroid use	0–1 courses/year	2–3 courses/year	> 3 courses/year

Adjust therapy

Down 1 step (if > 3 months)	Up 1 step[1] re-assess in 2–6 weeks	Up 1–2 steps[1,2] re-assess in 2 weeks

Preferred medical therapies	Steps in asthma management[3]					
	1	2[a]	3[b]	4[c,4]	5[d]	6[d,e]
Oral corticosteroids						▓
ICS-high potency					▓	▓
ICS-medium potency				▓		
ICS-low potency		▓	▓			
Long-acting bronchodilator			▓	▓	▓	▓
Short-acting bronchodilator	▓	▓	▓	▓	▓	▓

Patient education and environmental control at each step

ASTHMA MANAGEMENT ALGORITHM FOR ADOLESCENTS AND ADULTS (AGE ≥ 12 YEARS)
Source: NHLBI, 2007

Inhaled corticosteroid potencies				
	Puff dose, mcg	Low	Medium	High
Beclomethasone	42–84	80–240	240–480	>480
Budesonide	200	200–600	600–1200	>1200
Flunisolide	250	500–1000	1000–2000	>2000
Flunisolide HFA	80	320	320–640	>640
Fluticasone HFA	44, 110, 220	88–264	254–440	>440
Fluticasone DPI	50, 100, 250	100–300	300–500	>500
Mometasone DPI	220	200	400	>400
Triamcinolone	100	300–750	750–1500	>1500

[1] First assess adherence, environmental control, and comorbid conditions.

[2] Oral corticosteroid pulse therapy should be strongly considered.

[3] Consult with asthma specialist if Step 4 or higher.

[4] Consider subcutaneous allergen immunotherapy for patients who have allergic asthma.

[a] Alternative regimens include cromolyn, nedocromil, LTRA, or theophylline.

[b] Alternative regimens include ICS-low potency + either LTRA, theophylline, or zileuton.

[c] Alternative regimens include ICS-medium potency + either LTRA, theophylline, or zileuton.

[d] Consider omalizumab for patients with allergies.

[e] Consider adding LTRA, theophylline, or zileuton prior to starting oral corticosteroids, although this approach has not been studied in clinical trials.

SABA = short-acting beta-agonist; ICS = inhaled corticosteriod; LTRA = leukotriene receptor antagonist; HFA = hydrofluoroalkane; DPI = dry powder inhaler

ATRIAL FIBRILLATION: MANAGEMENT, PHARMACOLOGIC
Source: **American Heart Association/American College of Cardiology/European Society of Cardiology**

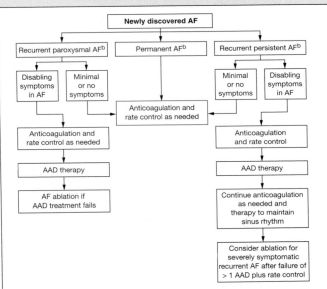

[a] Three objectives: rate control, prevention of thromboembolism, correction of rhythm disturbance (not mutually exclusive).

[b] Paroxysmal atrial fibrillation episodes last more than 30 seconds, but ≤ 7 days. If ≥ 2 episodes, designate "recurrent." When sustained > 7 days, designate "persistent."

Evidence update:

The AFFIRM trial showed no significant benefit of rhythm control (beyond rate control) in mortality or stroke risk and increased risk of death among older patients, those with congestive heart failure, and those with coronary disease. Rhythm control also increased hospitalization and adverse drug effects. (NEJM 2002;347:1825) Special considerations include patient symptoms, exercise tolerance, and patient preference. Current data do not support use of atrial pacing in the management of atrial fibrillation without symptomatic bradycardia. (Circulation 2005;111:240–243)

Non-valvular atrial fibrillation stroke risk calculation (JAMA 2001;285:2864–2870) CHADS2 = congestive heart failure, hypertension, age > 75 years, diabetes, and prior stroke or TIA. One point per factor, except 2 points for 2.5% per year. Low risk = score 0 or 1 = 1% per year. Moderate risk = score 2 = 2.5% per year. High risk = score 3 = 5% per year. All prior stroke or TIA should be considered high risk.

AF = atrial fibrillation; AAD = antiarrhythmic drug

Source: ACC/AHA/ESC, Circulation 2006;114:e257–e354.

ATRIAL FIBRILLATION: MANAGEMENT, ANTITHROMBOTIC THERAPY
Source: **American Heart Association/American College of Cardiology/European Society of Cardiology**

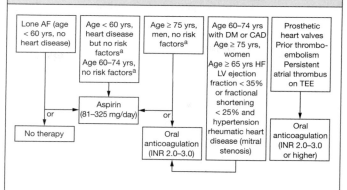

[a] Risk factors for thromboembolism: heart failure (HF), left ventricular ejection fraction < 35%, history of hypertension.

DM = diabetes mellitus; CAD = coronary artery disease; TEE = transesophageal echocardiography

Source: Circulation 2006;114:e257–e354.

ATRIAL FIBRILLATION: MANAGEMENT, ANTIARRHYTHMIC DRUG THERAPY
Source: American Heart Association/American College of Cardiology/European Society of Cardiology

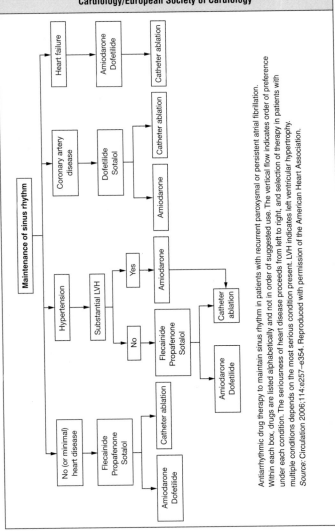

Antiarrhythmic drug therapy to maintain sinus rhythm in patients with recurrent paroxysmal or persistent atrial fibrillation. Within each box, drugs are listed alphabetically and not in order of suggested use. The vertical flow indicates order of preference under each condition. The seriousness of heart disease proceeds from left to right, and selection of therapy in patients with multiple conditions depends on the most serious condition present. LVH indicates left ventricular hypertrophy. *Source:* Circulation 2006;114:e257–e354. Reproduced with permission of the American Heart Association.

ATRIAL FIBRILLATION: MANAGEMENT, PHARMACOLOGIC AGENTS FOR RATE CONTROL
Source: American Heart Association/American College of Cardiology/European Society of Cardiology

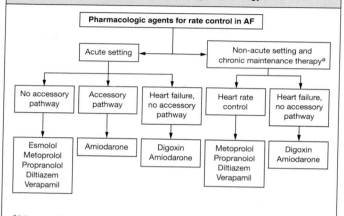

[a]Adequacy of heart rate control should be assessed during physical activity as well as at rest.

Source: Circulation 2006;114:e257–e354.

CANCER SURVIVORSHIP: LATE EFFECTS OF CANCER TREATMENTS

Cancer or Cancer Treatment History	Late Effect Type	Periodic Evaluation
Any cancer experience	Psychosocial disorders[b]	
Any chemotherapy	Oral and dental abnormalities	Dental exam and cleaning (every 6 months)
Chemotherapy (alkylating agents)[a]	Gonadal dysfunction	Pubertal assessment (yearly)
	Hematologic disorders[c]	History, exam for bleeding disorder; CBC/differential (yearly)
	Ocular toxicity[d]	Visual acuity, fundoscopic exam, evaluation by ophthalmologist (if radiation) (yearly if ocular tumors, TBI, or ≥ 30 Gy; else every 3 years)
	Pulmonary toxicity[e]	CXR, PFTs (at entry into long-term follow-up, then as clinically indicated)
	Renal toxicity[f]	Blood pressure (yearly); electrolytes, BUN, Cu, Ca^{++}, Mg^{++}, PO_4^-, urinalysis (at entry into long-term follow-up, then clinically as indicated)
	Urinary tract toxicity[g]	Urinalysis (yearly)
Chemotherapy (anthracycline antibiotics)[a]	Cardiac toxicity[h]	ECHO or MUGA, EKG at entry into long-term follow-up, periodic thereafter (↑ frequency if chest radiation); fasting glucose, lipid panel (every 3–5 years)
	Hematologic disorders[c]	See "chemotherapy (alkylating agents)"
Chemotherapy (bleomycin)[a]	Pulmonary toxicity[e]	See "chemotherapy (alkylating agents)"
Chemotherapy (cytarabine, high-dose IV; methotrexate, high-dose IV, IO, IT)	Clinical leukoencephalopathy[i] Neurocognitive deficits	Full neurologic exam (yearly) Neuropsychological evaluation (at entry into long-term follow-up, then as clinically indicated)
Chemotherapy (epipodophyllotoxins)[a]	Hematologic disorders[c]	See "chemotherapy (alkylating agents)"

CANCER SURVIVORSHIP: LATE EFFECTS OF CANCER TREATMENTS (CONTINUED)

Cancer or Cancer Treatment History	Late Effect Type	Periodic Evaluation
Chemotherapy (heavy metals)[a]	Dyslipidemia	Fasting lipid panel at entry
	Gonadal dysfunction	See "chemotherapy (alkylating agents)"
	Hematologic disorders[c]	See "chemotherapy (alkylating agents)"
	Ototoxicity[j]	Complete pure tone audiogram or brainstem auditory evoked response (yearly × 5 years, then every 5 years)
	Peripheral sensory neuropathy	Exam yearly for 2–3 years
	Renal toxicity[f]	See "chemotherapy (alkylating agents)"
Chemotherapy (methotrexate)	Osteopenia/osteoporosis	Bone density (at entry into long-term follow-up, then as clinically indicated)
	Renal toxicity[f]	See "chemotherapy (alkylating agents)"
Chemotherapy (non-classical alkylators)[a]	Gonadal dysfunction	See "chemotherapy (alkylating agents)"
	Hematologic disorders[c]	See "chemotherapy (alkylating agents)"
Chemotherapy (plant alkaloids)[a]	Peripheral sensory neuropathy	See "chemotherapy (heavy metals)"
	Raynaud's phenomenon	Yearly history/exam
Corticosteroids (dexamethasone, prednisone)	Ocular toxicity[d]	See "chemotherapy (alkylating agents)"
	Osteonecrosis	Musculoskeletal exam (yearly)
	Osteopenia/osteoporosis	See "chemotherapy (methotrexate)"

CANCER SURVIVORSHIP: LATE EFFECTS OF CANCER TREATMENTS (CONTINUED)

Cancer or Cancer Treatment History	Late Effect Type	Periodic Evaluation
Hematopoietic cell (bone marrow) transplant	Hematologic disorders[c]	See "chemotherapy (alkylating agents)"
	Oncologic disorders[k]	Inspection/exam targeted to irradiation fields (yearly)
	Osteonecrosis	See "chemotherapy (dexamethasone, prednisone)"
	Osteopenia/osteoporosis	See "chemotherapy (methotrexate)"
Radiation therapy (field- and dose-dependent)	Cardiac toxicity[h]	See "chemotherapy (alkylating agents)"
	Central adrenal insufficiency	8 AM serum cortisol (yearly × 15 years, and as clinically indicated)
	Cerebrovascular complications[l]	Neurologic exam (yearly)
	Chronic sinusitis	Head/neck exam (yearly)
	Functional asplenia	Blood culture when temperature ≥ 101°F
	Gonadal dysfunction	See "chemotherapy (alkylating agents)"
	Growth hormone deficiency	Height, weight, BMI (every 6 months until growth completed then yearly; Tanner staging (every 6 months until sexually mature)
	Hyperthyroidism	TSH, free T_4 (yearly)
	Hyperprolactinemia	Prolactin level (as clinically indicated)
	Hypothyroidism	TSH, free T_4
	Neurocognitive deficits	See "chemotherapy (cytarabine)"
	Ocular toxicity[d]	See "chemotherapy (alkylating agents)"
	Oncologic disorders[k]	See "hematopoietic cell (bone marrow) transplant"
	Oral and dental abnormalities	See "any chemotherapy"
	Ototoxicity[j]	See "chemotherapy (heavy metals)"
	Overweight/obesity/metabolic syndrome	Fasting glucose, fasting serum insulin, fasting lipid profile (every 2 years if overweight or obese; every 5 years if normal weight)

CANCER SURVIVORSHIP: LATE EFFECTS OF CANCER TREATMENTS (CONTINUED)

Cancer or Cancer Treatment History	Late Effect Type	Periodic Evaluation
	Pulmonary toxicity[e] Renal toxicity[f] Urinary tract toxicity[g]	See "chemotherapy (alkylating agents)" See "chemotherapy (alkylating agents)" See "chemotherapy (alkylating agents)"

[a]Chemotherapeutic agents, by class:
- Alkylating agents: Busulfan, carmustine (BCNU), chlorambucil, cyclophosphamide, ifosfamide, lomustine (CCNU), mechlorethamine, melphalan, procarbazine, thiotepa
- Heavy metals: Carboplatin, cisplatin
- Non-classical alkylators: Dacarbazine (DTIC), temozolomide
- Anthracycline antibiotics: Daunorubicin, doxorubicin, epirubicin, idarubicin, mitoxantrone
- Plant alkaloids: Vinblastine, vincristine
- Epipodophyllotoxins: Etoposide (VP16), teniposide (VM26)

[b]Psychosocial disorders: Mental health disorders, risky behaviors, psychosocial disability due to pain, fatigue, limitations in health care/insurance access.

[c]Hematologic disorders: Acute myeloid leukemia, myelodysplasia.

[d]Ocular toxicity: Cataracts, orbital hypoplasia, lacrimal duct atrophy, xerophthalmia, keratitis, telangiectasias, retinopathy, optic chiasm neuropathy, endophthalmos, chronic painful eye, maculopathy, papillopathy, glaucoma.

[e]Pulmonary toxicity: Pulmonary fibrosis, interstitial pneumonitis, restrictive lung disease, obstructive lung disease.

[f]Renal toxicity: Glomerular and tubular renal insufficiency, hypertension.

[g]Urinary tract toxicity: Hemorrhagic cystitis, bladder fibrosis, dysfunctional voiding, vesicoureteral reflux, hydronephrosis, bladder malignancy.

[h]Cardiac toxicity: Cardiomyopathy, arrhythmias, left ventricular dysfunction, congestive heart failure, pericarditis, pericardial fibrosis, valvular disease, myocardial infarction, atherosclerotic heart disease.

[i]Clinical leukoencephalopathy: Spasticity, ataxia, dysarthria, dysphagia, hemiparesis, seizures.

[j]Ototoxicity: Sensorineural hearing loss, tinnitus, vertigo, tympanosclerosis, otosclerosis, eustachian tube dysfunction, conductive hearing loss.

[k]Oncologic disorders: Secondary benign or malignant neoplasm.

[l]Cerebrovascular complications: Stroke, moyamoya, occlusive cerebral vasculopathy.

TBI = total body irradiation

Note: Guidelines for surveillance and monitoring for late effects after treatment for adult cancers available via the National Comprehensive Cancer Network, Inc. (NCCN) (http://www.nccn.org/professionals/physician_gls)

Source: Long-Term Follow-Up Guidelines for Survivors of Childhood, Adolescent, and Young Adult Cancers. Children's Oncology Group, Version 2.0, March 2006 (for full guidelines and references, see http://www.survivorshipguidelines.org).

See also: NEJM 2006;355:1722–1782.

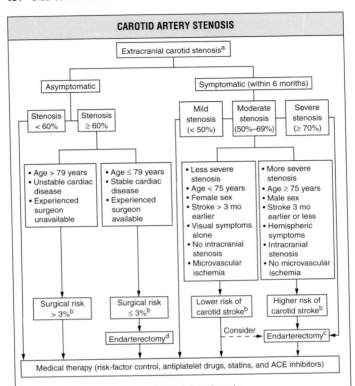

CAROTID ARTERY STENOSIS

Extracranial carotid stenosis[a]

Asymptomatic — Symptomatic (within 6 months)

Asymptomatic:
- Stenosis < 60%
- Stenosis ≥ 60%

Symptomatic:
- Mild stenosis (< 50%)
- Moderate stenosis (50%–69%)
- Severe stenosis (≥ 70%)

Stenosis ≥ 60%:
- Age > 79 years
- Unstable cardiac disease
- Experienced surgeon unavailable

- Age ≤ 79 years
- Stable cardiac disease
- Experienced surgeon available

Moderate:
- Less severe stenosis
- Age < 75 years
- Female sex
- Stroke > 3 mo earlier
- Visual symptoms alone
- No intracranial stenosis
- Microvascular ischemia

- More severe stenosis
- Age ≥ 75 years
- Male sex
- Stroke 3 mo earlier or less
- Hemispheric symptoms
- Intracranial stenosis
- No microvascular ischemia

Surgical risk > 3%[b]

Surgical risk ≤ 3%[b] → Endarterectomy[d]

Lower risk of carotid stroke[b]

Higher risk of carotid stroke[b] → Consider ---→ Endarterectomy[c]

Medical therapy (risk-factor control, antiplatelet drugs, statins, and ACE inhibitors)

[a]Best method for measuring degree of stenosis is angiography.

[b]Retrospective review of 1370 CEA (1990–1999) at 1 teaching hospital: no significant difference in incidence of perioperative stroke or death in those with ≥ 1 vs. no risk factors. 30-day mortality significantly greater (2.8% vs. 0.3%, p = 0.04) in those with ≥ 2 vs. no risk factors. (J Vasc Surg 2003;37:1191–1199)

[c]Surgery should generally be reserved for patients with > 5-year life expectancy and peri-operative stroke/death rate < 6% (AAN). When CEA is indicated, performance within 2 weeks is optimal.

[d]Given proven efficacy of CEA in healthy men with asymptomatic carotid stenosis > 60%, the only rational use of carotid angioplasty and stenting in this population is in the setting of randomized trials. [Stroke 2007;38(part 2):715–720]

Source: Adapted from The Guidelines of the American Heart Association, the American Stroke Association, and the American Academy of Neurology (2005). Other factors not included in the figure may also be relevant in risk stratification (eg, the results of cardiac evaluation or hemodynamic testing). Circulation 2006;113:e873. Stroke 2006;37:577.

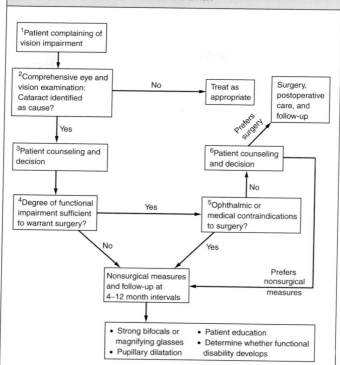

CATARACT IN ADULTS: EVALUATION & MANAGEMENT ALGORITHM
Source: AAO & AOA

Sources: American Academy of Ophthalmology Preferred Practice Pattern: Cataract in the
Adult Eye. (2006) (http://www.aao.org/PPP)
American Optometric Association Consensus Panel on Care of the Adult Patient with
Cataract. Optometric Clinical Practice Guideline: Care of the Adult Patient with Cataract.
(2004) (http://www.aoa.org)

Notes:

1. Begin evaluation only when patients complain of a vision problem or impairment. Identifying impairment in visual function during routine history and physical examination constitutes sound medical practice.

2. Essential elements of the comprehensive eye and vision examination:
   - *Patient history:* Consider cataract if: acute or gradual onset of vision loss; vision problems under special conditions (eg, low contrast, glare); difficulties performing various visual tasks. Ask about: refractive history, previous ocular disease, amblyopia, eye surgery, trauma, general health history, medications, and allergies. It is critical to describe the actual impact of the cataract on the person's function and quality of life. There are several instruments available for assessing functional impairment related to cataract, including VF-14, Activities of Daily Vision Scale, and Visual Activities Questionnaire.
   - *Ocular examination,* including: Snellen acuity and refraction; measurement of intraocular pressure; assessment of pupillary function; external examination; slit-lamp examination; and dilated examination of fundus.
   - *Supplemental testing:* May be necessary to assess and document the extent of the functional disability and to determine whether other diseases may limit preoperative or postoperative vision. Most elderly patients presenting with visual problems do not have a cataract that causes functional impairment. Refractive error, macular degeneration, and glaucoma are common alternative etiologies for visual impairment.

3. Once cataract has been identified as the cause of visual disability, patients should be counseled concerning the nature of the problem, its natural history, and the existence of both surgical and nonsurgical approaches to management. The principal factor that should guide decision making with regard to surgery is *the extent to which the cataract impairs the ability to function in daily life.* The findings of the physical examination should corroborate that the cataract is the major contributing cause of the functional impairment, and that there is a reasonable expectation that managing the cataract will positively impact the patient's functional activity. Preoperative visual acuity is a poor predictor of postoperative functional improvement: The decision to recommend cataract surgery should not be made solely on the basis of visual acuity.

4. Patients who complain of mild to moderate limitation in activities due to a visual problem, those whose corrected acuities are near 20/40, and those who do not yet wish to undergo surgery may be offered nonsurgical measures for improving visual function. Treatment with nutritional supplements is not recommended. Smoking cessation retards cataract progression. Indications for surgery: cataract-impaired vision no longer meets the patient's needs; evidence of lens-induced disease (eg, phakomorphic glaucoma, phakolytic glaucoma); necessary to visualize the fundus in an eye that has the potential for sight (eg, diabetic patient at risk of diabetic retinopathy).

5. *Contraindications to surgery:* the patient does not desire surgery; glasses or vision aids provide satisfactory functional vision; surgery will not improve visual function; the patient's quality of life is not compromised; the patient is unable to undergo surgery because of coexisting medical or ocular conditions; a legal consent cannot be obtained; or the patient is unable to obtain adequate postoperative care. Routine preoperative medical testing (12-lead EKG, CBC, measurement of serum electrolytes, BUN, creatinine, and glucose), while commonly performed in patients scheduled to undergo cataract surgery, does not appear to measurably increase the safety of the surgery.

6. Patients with significant functional and visual impairment due to cataract who have no contraindications to surgery should be counseled regarding the expected risks and benefits of and alternatives to surgery.

CHOLESTEROL & LIPID MANAGEMENT IN ADULTS
Source: NCEP, ATP III

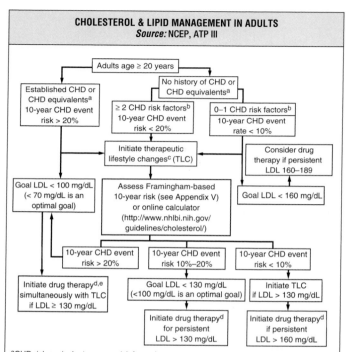

aCHD risk equivalents carry a risk for major coronary events equal to that of established CHD (ie, > 20% per 10 years), and include: diabetes, other clinical forms of atherosclerotic disease (peripheral arterial disease, abdominal aortic aneurysm, and symptomatic carotid artery disease).

bAge (men ≥ 45 years, women ≥ 55 years or postmenopausal), hypertension (BP ≥ 140/90 mm Hg or on antihypertensive medication), cigarette smoking, HDL < 40 mg/dL, family history of premature CHD in first-degree relative (males < 55 years, females < 65 years). For HDL ≥ 60 mg/dL, subtract 1 risk factor from above.

cReduce saturated fat (< 7% total calories) and cholesterol (< 200 mg/d intake); increase physical activity; and achieve appropriate weight control. Assess effects of TLC on lipid levels after 3 months.

dDrug therapy response should be monitored and modified at 6-week intervals to achieve goal LDL levels; after goal LDL met, monitor response and adherence every 4–6 months.

eAddition of fibrate or nicotinic acid is also an option if ↑ TGs or ↓ HDL.

Source: Executive summary of the third report of the National Cholesterol Education Project (NCEP) expert panel on detection, evaluation and treatment of high blood cholesterol in adults (Adult Treatment Panel III). JAMA 2001;285:2486. Implications of Recent Clinical Trials for the National Cholesterol Education Program Adult Treatment Panel III Guidelines. Circulation 2004;110:227–239

2004 MODIFICATIONS TO THE
ATP III TREATMENT ALGORITHM FOR LDL-C

In high-risk persons (10-year CHD risk > 20%), the recommended LDL-C goal is < 100 mg/dL.

An LDL-C goal of < 70 mg/dL is a therapeutic option, especially for patients at very high risk.

If LDL-C is ≥ 100 mg/dL, an LDL-lowering drug is indicated as initial therapy simultaneously with lifestyle changes.

If baseline LDL-C is < 100 mg/dL, institution of an LDL-lowering drug to achieve an LDL-C level < 70 mg/dL is a therapeutic option.

If a high-risk person has high triglycerides or low HDL-C, consideration can be given to combining a fibrate or nicotinic acid with an LDL-lowering drug. When triglycerides are ≥ 200 mg/dL, non–HDL-C is a secondary target of therapy, with a goal 30 mg/dL higher than the identified LDL-C goal.

For **moderately high-risk persons** (2+ risk factors and 10-year risk 10%–20%), the recommended LDL-C goal is < 130 mg/dL; an LDL-C goal < 100 mg/dL is a therapeutic option. When LDL-C level is 100–129 mg/dL, at baseline or on lifestyle therapy, initiation of an LDL-lowering drug to achieve an LDL-C level < 100 mg/dL is a therapeutic option.

Any person at high risk or moderately high risk who has lifestyle-related risk factors (eg, obesity, physical inactivity, elevated triglyceride, low HDL-C, or metabolic syndrome) is a candidate for TLC to modify these risk factors regardless of LDL-C level.

When LDL-lowering drug therapy is employed in high-risk or moderately high-risk persons, intensity of therapy should be sufficient to achieve at least a 30%–40% reduction in LDL-C levels.

Source: Implications of Recent Clinical Trials for the National Cholesterol Education Program Adult Treatment Panel III guidelines. Circulation 2004;110:227–239.

CHOLESTEROL & LIPID MANAGEMENT IN CHILDREN
Source: AHA, 2007

Children:
- Consider drug therapy if, after 6–12 month trial of fat- and cholesterol-restricted dietary management
  - LDL ≥ 190 mg/dL or
  - LDL > 160 mg/dL and postive family history of premature CHD; ≥ 2 other risk factors are present
- Treatment goal < 110 mg/dL (ideal) or < 130 mg/dL (minimal)
- Do not start before age 10 years in boys and until after menarche in girls
- Statins (HMG CoA reductase inhibitors) first-line drug therapy

Source: Circulation 2007;115:1948–1967.

COPD MANAGEMENT: STABLE COPD
Source: Adapted from ATS/ERS and GOLD Initiative, 2006

GOLD classification based on FEV, when FEV/FVC < 0.70

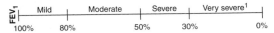

Pharmacologic therapy

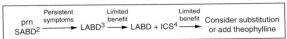

Indications for home oxygen

Based on waking O_2 at sea level
- $PaO_2 \le 55$ mm Hg or O_2 saturation $\le 88\%$
- $PaO_2 \le 60$ mm Hg if cor pulmonale, peripheral edema, or polycythemia (Hct > 55%)

Target O_2: $PaO_2 = 60$ mm Hg or O_2 saturation = 90%

Indications for lung volume reduction surgery

- FEV = 20%–45%
- Upper lobe emphysema and low exercise capacity despite medical therapy

Indications for lung transplant

- Advanced lung disease with high risk of death in 2–3 years
- Lack of success of alternative therapies
- Severe functional limitation, but preserved ability to walk
- Age ≤ 55 years (heart–lung transplant); ≤ 60 years (bilateral lung transplant); ≤ 65 years (single lung transplant)

Pulmonary rehabilitation

- Exercise training
- Strength training
- Education
- Psychosocial and behavioral support
- Nutritional counseling

[1] Very severe also appropriate when $FEV_1 < 50\%$ plus chronic respiratory failure ($PaO_2 < 60$ mm Hg or $PCO_2 > 50$ mm Hg breathing room air at sea level).

[2] SABD: Short-acting bronchodilators, beta$_2$-agonist or anticholinergic metered-dose inhalers.

[3] LABD: Long-acting bronchodilators, such as salmeterol or tiotropium.

[4] ICS: inhaled corticosteroid. Combination LABD and ICS supported in NEJM 2007;356:775. Combination ICS-salmeterol plus tiotropium improved lung function and quality of life. (Ann Intern Med 2007;146:545)

Source: http://www.goldcopd.com

COPD MANAGEMENT: COPD EXACERBATION
Source: ATS/ERS

	Level I	Level II	Level III
Clinical history			
Co-morbid conditions#	+	+++	+++
History of frequent exacerbations	+	+++	+++
Severity of COPD	Mild/moderate	Moderate/severe	Severe
Physical findings			
Hemodynamic evaluation	Stable	Stable	Stable/unstable
Use accessory respiratory muscles, tachypnea	Not present	++	+++
Persistent symptoms after initial therapy	No	++	+++
Diagnostic procedures			
Oxygen saturation	Yes	Yes	Yes
Arterial blood gases	No	Yes	Yes
Chest radiograph	No	Yes	Yes
Blood tests¶	No	Yes	Yes
Serum drug concentrations+	If applicable	If applicable	If applicable
Sputum gram stain and culture	No§	Yes	Yes
Electrocardiogram	No	Yes	Yes

+: unlikely to be present; ++: likely to be present; +++: very likely to be present.
#: the more common co-morbid conditions associated with poor prognosis in exacerbations are congestive heart failure, coronary artery disease, diabetes mellitus, renal and liver failure; ¶: blood tests include cell blood count, serum electrolytes, renal and liver function; +: serum drug concentrations, consider if patients are using theophylline, warfarin, carbamezepine, digoxin; §: consider if patient has recently been on antibiotics.

Level I: Outpatient Treatment

Patient education
  Check inhalation technique
  Consider use of spacer devices
Bronchodilators
  Short-acting β_2-agonist# and/or ipratropium MDI with spacer or hand-held nebulizer as needed
  Consider adding long-acting bronchodilator if patient is not using one
Corticosteroids (the actual dose may vary)
  Prednisone 30–40 mg orally·day^{-1} for 10–14 days
  Consider using an inhaled corticosteroid
Antibiotics
  May be initiated in patients with altered sputum characteristics+
  Choice should be based on local bacterial resistance patterns
  Amoxicillin/ampicillin¶, cephalosporins
  Doxycycline
  Macrolides§
  If the patient has failed prior antibiotic therapy consider: amoxicillin/clavulanate; respiratory fluoroquinolones^f

Level II: Hospitalization Treatment

Bronchodilators
  Short-acting β_2-agonist and/or Ipratropium MDI with hand-held nebulizer as needed
Supplemental oxygen (if saturation < 90%)
Corticosteroids
  If patient tolerates, prednisone 30–40 mg orally·day^{-1} for 10–14 days
  If patient cannot tolerate oral intake, equivalent dose IV for up to 14 days
  Consider using inhaled corticosteroids by MDI or hand-held nebulizer
Antibiotics (based on local bacterial resistance patterns)
  May be initiated in patients that have a change in their sputum characteristics+
  Choice should be based on local bacterial resistance patterns
  Amoxicillin/clavulanate
  Respiratory fluoroquinolones (gatifloxacin, levofloxacin, moxifloxacin)
  If Pseudomonas spp. and/or other Enterobacteriaceae spp. are suspected, consider combination therapy

MDI: metered-dose inhaler. #: salbutamol (albuterol), terbutaline; +: purulence and/or volume; ¶: depending on local prevalence of bacterial β-lactamases; §: azithromycin, clarithromycin, dirithromycin, roxithromycin; f: gatifloxacin, levofloxacin, moxifloxacin.
Source: Eur Resp J 2004;23:932–946.

MDI: metered-dose inhaler. #: purulence and/or volume.
Source: Celli B, et al. Standards for the diagnosis and treatment of patients with COPD: a summary of the ATS-ERS position paper. Eur Respir J 2004;23:932–946.

CORONARY ARTERY DISEASE
Post-Myocardial Infarction Risk Stratification[a]

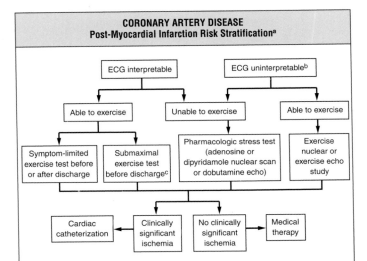

Modified from: ACC/AHA Guidelines for the Management of Patients with ST-Elevation Myocardial Infarction. Circulation 2004;110:588–636.

[a]Risk stratification occurs after acute management of ST-elevation myocardial infarction.

[b]Patient on digoxin, baseline left bundle branch block or left ventricular hypertrophy.

[c]If strenuous leisure activity or occupation, perform symptom-limited exercise testing at 3–6 weeks to confirm.

Note: Per ACC/AHA guidelines, all patients age ≥ 70 years are at intermediate risk and patients age ≥ 75 years are at high risk for short-term death or non-fatal MI. (Circulation 2007;115:2549–2569)

AHA "Get with the Guidelines" program is a web-based program to help hospitals improve quality of care for coronary artery disease, and provide real-time benchmarking of performance and quality measures. (http://americanheart.org/getwiththeguidelines)

DEPRESSION: ASSESSMENT
Source: Adapted from Colorado Clinical Guidelines Collaborative, 2006

MAJOR DEPRESSION DISORDER IN ADULTS (PART I): DIAGNOSIS

Common Symptoms
- Pains and aches
- Low energy
- Apathy, irritability, anxiety, sadness
- Sexual complaints
- Disrupted sleep patterns
- Vague GI symptoms
- Concentration difficulties

High-Risk Conditions
- Chronic disease
- ETOH/substance abuse
- Chronic pain
- Postpartum
- Victim of abuse/trauma

Attend to common symptoms of depression during routine medical screens (PHQ-9 highly recommended as screening tool)

Depression Criteria (DSM IV): 5 or more in same 2 weeks, including at least one of the first two symptoms
- Depressed mood
- Marked diminished interest/pleasure
- Significant weight gain or loss
- Insomnia or hypersomnia
- Psychomotor agitation or retardation
- Fatigue or loss of energy
- Feelings of worthlessness or inappropriate guilt
- Diminished concentration or indecisiveness
- Suicidal ideation (thoughts, plans, means, intent)

If imminently suicidal, consider psych consult, emergency hold, 911, and/or psychiatric inpatient evaluation.

Confirm diagnosis using criteria and/or depression scale

Consider Comorbid Medical Psychiatric Disorders
Carefully screen for bipolar and substance abuse

Continued on next page

Treatment and/or Referral Options:
- **Medications**—*especially for moderate to severe and/or chronic symptoms*
- **Referral to Outpatient Psychotherapy**—suitable for *mild* to *moderate* symptoms
- **Combined** medication and psychotherapy—for more *severe* symptoms and incomplete response to either medications or therapy

Determine method of treatment
- Medication
- Psychotherapy
- Both

Medication Selection and Dosage Considerations:
- Existing medical and psychiatric conditions
- Side effects
- Lethality for suicidal patients

Educate patient about:
- medication side effects
- importance of compliance
- not character defect/personal weakness

DEPRESSION: TREATMENT
Source: **Adapted from Colorado Clinical Guidelines Collaborative, 2006**

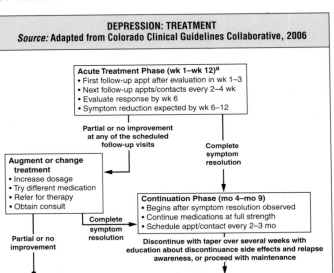

Acute Treatment Phase (wk 1–wk 12)[a]
- First follow-up appt after evaluation in wk 1–3
- Next follow-up appts/contacts every 2–4 wk
- Evaluate response by wk 6
- Symptom reduction expected by wk 6–12

Partial or no improvement at any of the scheduled follow-up visits

Complete symptom resolution

Augment or change treatment
- Increase dosage
- Try different medication
- Refer for therapy
- Obtain consult

Continuation Phase (mo 4–mo 9)
- Begins after symptom resolution observed
- Continue medications at full strength
- Schedule appt/contact every 2–3 mo

Complete symptom resolution

Discontinue with taper over several weeks with education about discontinuance side effects and relapse awareness, or proceed with maintenance

Partial or no improvement

Obtain psych consult or refer to mental health specialty care[b]

Maintenance Phase (mo 9 and on)
- At-risk for relapse based on history or genetic disposition
- Aimed at preventing relapse
- Continue medications for 1 to several years

[a] • Monitor for increased anxiety/agitation with suicidal ideation
- Monitor for onset of mania (see Mood Disorder Questionnaire at http://www.psycheducation.org/depression/MDQ.htm)
- Monitor treatment response using depression scale (PHQ-9) and/or DSM-IV criteria
- Ongoing patient education on course of illness and compliance

[b] **Psych Consult/Referral Considerations**
- Psychotic/bipolar/severe depressive state
- Active suicidal, homicidal, self-injurious behavior
- Co-existing substance abuse/dependence
- Specialized treatment for psychotic/severe depression (eg, ECT)
- Ongoing monitoring indicates decline
- Partial or no response to one or more medication trials
- Complex psychological issues
- Co-administering second psychotropic medication
- Medically unstable geriatric patient
- Second opinion desired
- Guideline not suitable for patient
- Administering antidepressant in pregnant woman

DEPRESSION: TREATMENT (CONTINUED)

Source: Reproduced, with permission, from Colorado Clinic Guidelines Collaborative. For references, medical record tracking forms, and long form, go to http://www.coloradoguidelines.org.

ACP guidelines recommend either tricyclic antidepressants or newer antidepressants, such as selective serotonin reuptake inhibitors, as equally efficacious. (Ann Intern Med 2000;132:738)

Treating depression effectively leads to improved comorbidity-associated pain control and functional status (eg, arthritis, diabetes). (JAMA 2003;290:2428; Ann Intern Med 2004;140:1015)

A trial using depression algorithms and depression care managers in older adults (age > 60) showed ↓ suicidal ideation and ↓ depression compared with usual care. (JAMA 2004;291:1081)

NCQA HEDIS Antidepression medication management measures:
  Optimum Practitioner Contact: Percent who received ≥ 3 follow-up office visits in the 12-week acute treatment phase after a new depression diagnosis
  Effective Acute Phase Treatment: Percent who received antidepressant medication in the 12-week acute treatment phase after new depression diagnosis
  Effective Continuation Phase Treatment: Percent who remained on antidepressant medication continuously for 6 months after initial diagnosis

DIABETES MELLITUS: MANAGEMENT

METABOLIC MANAGEMENT OF TYPE 2 DIABETES
Source: ADA AND EUROPEAN ASSOCIATION FOR THE STUDY OF DIABETES

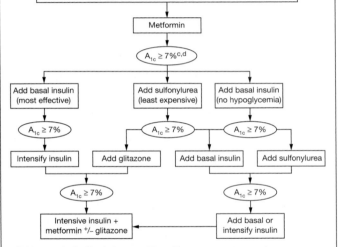

^{a}Diabetes = fasting blood glucose ≥ 126 mg/dL on two separate occasions, or symptoms of diabetes with random glucose ≥ 200 mg/dL.

^{b}Reinforce lifestyle intervention at every visit.

^{c}Treatment goals: A_{1c} < 7%; fasting and preprandial blood glucose 70–130 mg/dL. These are generalized goals. They do not apply to pregnant women. Modify individual treatment goals taking into account risk for hypoglycemia, very young or old age, end-stage renal disease, advanced cardiovascular or cerebrovascular disease, and life expectancy.

^{d}Check A_{1c} every 3 months until < 7% and then at least every 6 months.

Source: Diabetes Care 2006;29:1963–2006.

PREVENTION & TREATMENT OF DIABETIC COMPLICATIONS/COMORBIDITIES
Source: ADA

Complication or Comorbidity	Goal	Monitoring/Treatment	Action If Goal Not Met
Hyperglycemia[a]	$HbA_{1c} < 7.0\%$[b] Preprandial plasma glucose 90–130 mg/dL Peak postprandial plasma glucose < 180 mg/dL	HbA_{1c} = every 6 months if meeting treatment goals; every 3 months in those not meeting goals or whose therapy has changed.	See management, previous page.
Retinopathy	Prevent vision loss	Optimize glycemic and blood pressure control. Annual retinal exam.[c]	Laser treatment.
Neuropathy	Prevent foot complications	Annual foot exam[d] and visual inspection at every visit.	Refer high-risk patients to a foot care specialist.
Nephropathy	Prevent renal failure	Optimize glucose and blood pressure control. Annual serum creatinine and microalbuminuria determination (see page 140). Spot urinoalbumin: creatinine testing preferred. Continued surveillance even if treated with ACE or ARB. Annual GFR calculation.[f] Limit protein intake to 0.8 g/kg in those with any degree of chronic kidney disease.	See below[e] for treatment; consider nephrology referral.
Hypertension	Adult: BP ≤ 130/80 mm Hg[g]	Measure at every routine diabetes visit.[h]	See JNC VII, page 142. If ACEs or adrenergic receptor binders are used, monitor renal function and potassium levels.

PREVENTION & TREATMENT OF DIABETIC COMPLICATIONS/COMORBIDITIES
Source: ADA

PREVENTION & TREATMENT OF DIABETIC COMPLICATIONS/COMORBIDITIES (CONTINUED)

Complication or Comorbidity	Goal	Monitoring/Treatment	Action If Goal Not Met
Hyperlipidemia	LDL < 100 mg/dL[i] TG < 150 mg/dL HDL > 40 mg/dL	Annual determination, and more frequently to achieve goals. If low-risk (LDL < 100, HDL > 60, TG < 150), then assess every 2 years. Routine monitoring of liver and muscle enzymes in asymptomatic patients is not recommended unless patient has baseline enzyme abnormalities or is taking drugs that interact with statins. (ACP: Ann Intern Med 2004;140:644)	Weight loss; increase in physical activity; nutrition therapy; follow NCEP recommendations for pharmacologic treatment, pages 127–128.
Macrovascular disease	Prevent limb ischemia, stroke, and MI	1. Use aspirin therapy (75–162 mg/day) as primary prevention for all patients ≥ 40 years or those with ≥ 1 cardiovascular risk factor. 2. Smoking cessation. 3. Manage hyperlipidemia and hypertension as above. 4. Assess for peripheral arterial disease with pedal pulses ± ankle brachial pressure index via doppler. 5. Consider ACE inhibitor if age > 55 years, with or without hypertension, if cardiovascular risk factor present.	Use aspirin as secondary prevention if history of MI, vascular bypass procedure, stroke or TIA, peripheral vascular disease, claudication, and/or angina.

PREVENTION & TREATMENT OF DIABETIC COMPLICATIONS/COMORBIDITIES
Source: ADA

PREVENTION & TREATMENT OF DIABETIC COMPLICATIONS/COMORBIDITIES (CONTINUED)

[a] Less intensive glycemic goals if severe or frequent hypoglycemia.

[b] Postprandial glucose may be targeted if HbA$_{1c}$ goals are not met despite meeting preprandial goals.

[c] Dilated eye exam or 7-field 30-degree fundus photography by ophthalmologist or optometrist. In setting of normal eye exam, less frequent screening can be considered by eye specialist.

[d] Includes evaluation of protective sensation (monofilament test and tuning fork), vascular status, and inspection for foot deformities or ulcers.

[e] Microalbuminuria treatment: if type 1, use ACE inhibitor; if type 2 and hypertensive, use ACE or ARB. Clinical albuminuria treatment: (1) Achieve BP < 130/80 mm Hg; (2) use ACE inhibitor or ARB; (3) tight glycemic control; and (4) decrease protein to 10% of dietary intake, especially in patients progressing despite optimal glucose and BP control. Refer to nephrologist if: estimated glomerular filtration rate < 30 mg/minute, creatinine > 2.0 mg/dL, or when management of hypertension or hyperkalemia is difficult.

[f] Estimated GFR calculator: http://www.kidney.org/professionals/kdoqi/gfr_calculator.cfm

[g] ALLHAT trial showed no difference in cardiovascular and renal outcomes in diabetes treated with diuretics or ACE (or ARB). (JAMA 2002;288:2981) Diuretics should be first line in black patients. (Ann Intern Med 2003;138:587)

[h] ACP recommends tight BP control (SBP < 135, DBP < 80).

[i] LDL < 70 mg/dL, using a high-dose statin, is an option in high-risk patients with DM and overt CVD.

Source: Adapted from American Diabetes Association Position Statement "Standards of Medical Care in Diabetes Mellitus 2007." Diabetes Care 2007;30(Suppl 1). Adult Diabetes." (2005) (http://www.nationaldiabetesalliance.org)

For recommended quality improvement and public reporting measures, see "National Diabetes Quality Improvement Alliance Performance Measurement Set for

For children (AHA): Circulation 2006;114:2710–2738.

For older adults (AGS): J Am Geriatr Society 2003;51(Suppl):S265–S280.

PREVENTION & TREATMENT OF DIABETIC COMPLICATIONS/COMORBIDITIES
Source: ADA

PREVENTION & TREATMENT OF DIABETIC COMPLICATIONS/COMORBIDITIES: KIDNEY DISEASE

Category[b]	Albuminuria Thresholds[a]		
	24-hour collection (mg/24 hour)	Timed collection (μg/minute)	Spot collection (albumin: creatinine ratio) (μg/mg)
Normal	< 30	< 20	< 30
Microalbuminuria	30–299	20–200	30–299
Clinical (macro) albuminuria	≥ 300	> 200	≥ 300

[a]Because of variability in urinary albumin excretion, 2 of 3 specimens collected within a 3- to 6-month period should be abnormal before considering a patient to have crossed one of these diagnostic thresholds. Exercise within 24 hours, infection, fever, congestive heart failure, marked hyperglycemia, and marked hypertension may elevate urinary albumin excretion over baseline values.

[b]Timed urine and 24-hr collections are rarely necessary. Spot collection is encouraged as the preferred test.

Source: ADA Diabetes Care 2007;30(Suppl 1).

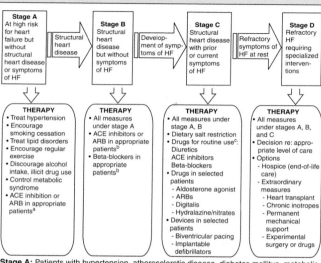

HEART FAILURE
Source: ACC/AHA, 2005

Stage A: Patients with hypertension, atherosclerotic disease, diabetes mellitus, metabolic syndrome, *or* those using cardiotoxins or having a FHx CM

Stage B: Patients with previous MI, LV remodeling including LVH and low EF, or asymptomatic valvular disease

Stage C: Patients with known structural heart disease; shortness of breath and fatigue, reduced exercise tolerance

Stage D: Patients who have marked symptoms at rest despite maximal medical therapy (eg, those who are recurrently hospitalized or cannot be safely discharged from hospital without specialized interventions)

Footnotes:
[a]History of atherosclerotic vascular disease, diabetes mellitus, or hypertension and associated cardiovascular risk factors.
[b]Recent or remote MI, regardless of ejection fraction; or reduced ejection fraction regardless of MI Hx. Use ARB in patients post-MI who cannot tolerate ACE inhibitors.
[c]Recent evidence suggests that isosorbide dinitrate plus hydralazine reduces mortality in blacks with advanced heart failure. (NEJM 2004;351:2049)

Comments: 1) Exercise training in patients with HF seems to be safe and beneficial overall in improving exercise capacity, quality of life, muscle structure, and physiologic responses to exercise. (Circulation 2003;107:1210–1225)

FHx CM = family history of cardiomyopathy; HF = heart failure; LV = left ventricle

Source: Adapted and reproduced with permission from the American College of Cardiology and American Heart Association, Inc. Circulation 2005;112:154–235.

AHA "Get with the Guidelines" program is a web-based program to help hospitals improve the quality of care for heart failure. Provides real-time benchmarking of performance and quality measures. (http://americanheart.org/getwiththeguidelines)

HYPERTENSION: INITIATING TREATMENT
Source: The 7th Report of the Joint National Committee
on Prevention, Detection, Evaluation, and Treatment of High
Blood Pressure, 2003

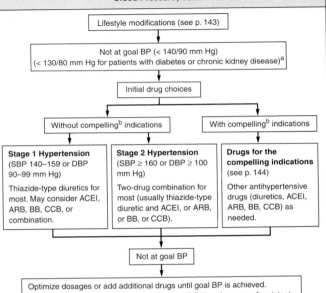

Lifestyle modifications (see p. 143)

Not at goal BP (< 140/90 mm Hg)
(< 130/80 mm Hg for patients with diabetes or chronic kidney disease)[a]

Initial drug choices

Without compelling[b] indications | With compelling[b] indications

Stage 1 Hypertension
(SBP 140–159 or DBP
90–99 mm Hg)

Thiazide-type diuretics for
most. May consider ACEI,
ARB, BB, CCB, or
combination.

Stage 2 Hypertension
(SBP ≥ 160 or DBP ≥ 100
mm Hg)

Two-drug combination for
most (usually thiazide-type
diuretic and ACEI, or ARB,
or BB, or CCB).

**Drugs for the
compelling indications**
(see p. 144)

Other antihypertensive
drugs (diuretics, ACEI,
ARB, BB, CCB) as
needed.

Not at goal BP

Optimize dosages or add additional drugs until goal BP is achieved.
Consider consultation with hypertension specialist, and causes of resistant
hypertension (see p. 145).

Drug abbreviations: ACEI, ACE inhibitor; ARB, angiotensin receptor blocker; BB,
beta-blocker; CCB, calcium channel blocker.

[a]AHA also recommends BP < 130/80 for patients with known CHD, carotid artery
disease, peripheral arterial disease, abdominal aortic aneurysm, or 10-year
Framingham risk score ≥ 10%; and BP < 120/80 for patients with left ventricular
dysfunction. (Circulation 2007;115:2761–2788)

[b]Compelling indications: CHF, high coronary disease risk, diabetes, chronic kidney
disease, recurrent stroke prevention, post MI.

Source: JNC VII, 2003. (Hypertension 2003;42:1206–1252)

Note: Cochrane review (2007): Available evidence does not support use of BB as
first-line drugs in treatment of hypertension. BB were inferior to CCB, renin-
angiotensin system inhibitors, and thiazide diuretics (although most trials used
atenolol). [Cochrane Database of Systematic Reviews 2007, Issue 1 (CD002003),
http://www.cochrane.org]

LIFESTYLE MODIFICATIONS FOR PRIMARY PREVENTION OF HYPERTENSION[a,b]

Modification	Recommendation	Approximate SBP Reduction (Range)
Weight reduction	Maintain normal body weight (BMI 18.5–24.9 kg/m^2).	5–20 mm Hg per 10 kg weight loss
Adopt DASH eating plan	Consume diet rich in fruits, vegetables, and low-fat dairy products with a reduced content of saturated and total fat.	8–14 mm Hg
Dietary sodium reduction	Reduce dietary sodium intake to no more than 100 mmol/day (2.4 g sodium or 6 g sodium chloride).	2–8 mm Hg
Physical activity	Engage in regular aerobic physical activity such as brisk walking (at least 30 min/day, most days of the week).	4–9 mm Hg
Moderation of alcohol consumption	Limit consumption to no more than 2 drinks (1 oz or 30 mL ethanol; eg, 24 oz beer, 10 oz wine, or 3 oz 80-proof whiskey) per day in most men and to no more than 1 drink per day in women and lighter-weight persons.	2–4 mm Hg

[a]For overall cardiovascular risk reduction, stop smoking.
[b]The effects of implementing these modifications are dose and time dependent and could be greater for some individuals.
DASH = Dietary Approaches to Stop Hypertension

RECOMMENDED MEDICATIONS FOR COMPELLING INDICATIONS

Compelling Indication[b]	Recommended Medications[a]					
	Diuretic	BB	ACEI	ARB	CCB	AldoANT
Heart failure	X	X	X	X		X
Post-MI		X	X			X
High coronary disease risk	X	X	X		X	
Diabetes	X	X	X	X	X	
Chronic kidney disease[c]			X	X		
Recurrent stroke prevention	X		X			

[a]Drug abbreviations: ACEI, ACE inhibitor; ARB, angiotensin receptor blocker; AldoANT, aldosterone antagonist; BB, beta-blocker; CCB, calcium channel blocker.
[b]Compelling indications for antihypertensive drugs are based on benefits from outcome studies or existing clinical guidelines; the compelling indication is managed in parallel with the BP.
[c]ALLHAT: Patients with hypertension and reduced GFR: No difference in renal outcomes (development of ESRD and/or decrement in GFR of $\geq$ 50% from baseline) comparing amlodipine, lisinopril, and chlorthalidone. [Arch Intern Med 2005 Apr 25;165(8):936–946]

HYPERTENSION: CHILDREN AND ADOLESCENTS

INDICATIONS FOR ANTIHYPERTENSIVE DRUG THERAPY IN CHILDREN AND ADOLESCENTS

- Symptomatic hypertension
- Secondary hypertension
- Hypertensive target organ damage
- Diabetes (types 1 and 2)
- Persistent hypertension despite non-pharmacologic measures (weight management counseling if overweight; physical activity; diet management)

Sources: Pediatrics 2004;114:555–576 and Circulation 2006;2710–2738.

CAUSES OF RESISTANT HYPERTENSION
Improper BP measurement
Volume overload and pseudotolerance
Excess sodium intake
Volume retention from kidney disease
Inadequate diuretic therapy
Drug-induced or other causes
Nonadherence
Inadequate doses
Inappropriate combinations
Nonsteroidal anti-inflammatory drugs; cyclooxygenase-2 inhibitors
Cocaine, amphetamines, other illicit drugs
Sympathomimetics (decongestants, anoretics)
Oral contraceptives
Adrenal steroids
Cyclosporine and tacrolimus
Erythropoietin
Licorice (including some chewing tobacco)
Over-the-counter dietary supplements and medicines (eg, ephedra, mahuang, bitter orange)
Associated conditions
Obesity
Excess alcohol intake
Identifiable causes
Sleep apnea
Chronic kidney disease
Primary aldosteronism
Renovascular disease
Steroid excess (Cushing's syndrome; chronic steroid therapy)
Pheochromocytoma
Coarctation of aorta
Thyroid or parathyroid disease
Obstructive uropathy

METABOLIC SYNDROME: IDENTIFICATION AND MANAGEMENT
Source: NCEP, ATP III, 2005

Clinical Identification

Risk Factor	Defining Level[a]
Abdominal obesity (waist circumference)[b]	
Men	> 102 cm (> 40 in.)
Women	> 88 cm (> 35 in.)
Triglycerides	≥ 150 mg/dL
HDL cholesterol	
Men	< 40 mg/dL
Women	< 50 mg/dL
Blood pressure	≥ 135/≥ 85 mm Hg
Fasting glucose	≥ 100 mg/dL

Management

- First-line therapy: Lifestyle modification leading to weight reduction and increased physical activity.
- Goal: ↓ Body weight by ~7%–10% over 6–12 months.
- At least 30 minutes of daily moderate-intensity physical activity.
- Low intake of saturated fats, trans fats, and cholesterol.
- Reduced consumption of simple sugars.
- Increased intake of fruits, vegetables, and whole grains.
- Avoid extremes in intake of either carbohydrates or fats.
- Smoking cessation.
- Drug therapy for hypertension, elevated LDL cholesterol, and diabetes.
- Consider combination therapy with fibrates or nicotinic acid plus a statin.
- Low-dose ASA for patients at intermediate and high risk.
- Bariatric surgery for BMI > 35 mg/kg^2.
- Clinical utility of identifying metabolic syndrome remains unclear as does not significantly add to the prediction of CHD risk compared to Framingham risk score. Recommended treatments are the same as those recommended for the individual risk factors. (JAMA 2006;295:819–821)

[a]NCEP ATP III definition (Circulation 2005;112:2735–2752)—Requires any 3 of the listed components.
[b]Waist circumference can identify persons at greater cardiometabolic risk than are identified by BMI alone. However, further studies needed to establish waist circumference cutpoints that assess risk not adequately captured by BMI. (Am J Clin Nutr 2007;85:1197–1202)
Note: World Health Organization (WHO) and International Diabetes Federation (IDF, http://www.idf.org) define metabolic syndrome slightly differently. There is no official definition of metabolic syndrome in children, but constellation of conditions confers significant increased risk of CHD. (Circulation 2007;115:1948–1967)

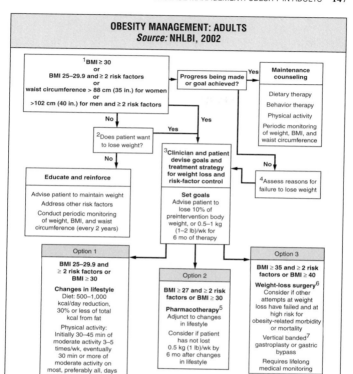

OBESITY MANAGEMENT: ADULTS
Source: NHLBI, 2002

[1]BMI ≥ 30
or
BMI 25–29.9 and ≥ 2 risk factors
or
waist circumference > 88 cm (35 in.) for women
or
>102 cm (40 in.) for men and ≥ 2 risk factors

→ Progress being made or goal achieved? —Yes→ **Maintenance counseling**

Dietary therapy
Behavior therapy
Physical activity
Periodic monitoring of weight, BMI, and waist circumference

No ↓ | Yes ↑

[2]Does patient want to lose weight? —Yes→

No ↓

Educate and reinforce

Advise patient to maintain weight
Address other risk factors
Conduct periodic monitoring of weight, BMI, and waist circumference (every 2 years)

[3]Clinician and patient devise goals and treatment strategy for weight loss and risk-factor control

Set goals
Advise patient to lose 10% of preintervention body weight, or 0.5–1 kg (1–2 lb)/wk for 6 mo of therapy

No → [4]Assess reasons for failure to lose weight

Option 1

BMI 25–29.9 and ≥ 2 risk factors or BMI ≥ 30

Changes in lifestyle
Diet: 500–1,000 kcal/day reduction, 30% or less of total kcal from fat
Physical activity: Initially 30–45 min of moderate activity 3–5 times/wk, eventually 30 min or more of moderate activity on most, preferably all, days
Behavior therapy

Option 2

BMI ≥ 27 and ≥ 2 risk factors or BMI ≥ 30

Pharmacotherapy[5]
Adjunct to changes in lifestyle
Consider if patient has not lost 0.5 kg (1 lb)/wk by 6 mo after changes in lifestyle

Option 3

BMI ≥ 35 and ≥ 2 risk factors or BMI ≥ 40

Weight-loss surgery[6]
Consider if other attempts at weight loss have failed and at high risk for obesity-related morbidity or mortality
Vertical banded[7] gastroplasty or gastric bypass
Requires lifelong medical monitoring

Notes for Obesity Management Guideline: Adults

1. <u>Risk factors</u>: cigarette smoking; hypertension or current use of antihypertensive agents; LDL cholesterol ≥ 160 mg/dL or LDL cholesterol 130–159 mg/dL + ≥ 2 other risk factors; HDL cholesterol < 35 mg/dL; fasting plasma glucose 110–125 mg/dL; family history of premature CHD (MI or sudden death in 1st degree ♂ relative ≤ 55 years old or 1st degree ♀ relative ≤ 65 years old; age ≥ 45 for ♂ or ≥ 55 years for ♀.
2. The decision to lose weight must be made in the context of other risk factors (eg, quitting smoking is more important than losing weight).
3. The decision to lose weight must be made jointly between the clinician and the patient.
4. <u>Investigate</u>: patient's level of motivation; energy intake (dietary recall); energy expenditure (physical activity diary); attendance at psychological/behavioral counseling sessions; recent negative life events; family and societal pressures; evidence of detrimental psychiatric problems (eg, depression, binge eating disorder).
5. Weight loss drugs may be used only as a part of a comprehensive weight loss program. Use for BMI ≥ 30 with no obesity-related risk factors or diseases and for BMI ≥ 27 with obesity-related risk factors or diseases. Options: bupropion, diethylproprion, fluoxetine, orlistat, phentermine, rimonabant, sibutramine. Data available past 12 months only for orlistat. (See Ann Intern Med 2005;142:525–531 and Gastroenterology 2007;132:2239–2252)
6. Refer to high-volume centers with surgeons experienced in bariatric surgery. 2007 review article: NEJM 2007;356:2176–2183.
7. Recent RCT showed 2-year outcome for laparoscopic gastric banding was superior to intensive medical (orlistat) and behavioral therapy (Ann Intern Med 2006;144:625–633).
Source: Adapted from the National Institutes of Health. NEJM 2002;346(8):591–599; http://www.nhlbi. nih.gov/guidelines/obesity/ob_home.htm

OBESITY MANAGEMENT: CHILDREN
Source: Expert Committee, Department of Health and Human Services

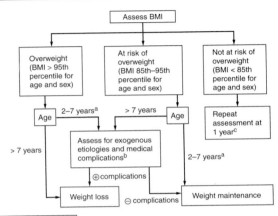

Approach to therapy:

1. Establish individual treatment goals and approaches based on child's age, degree of overweight, presence of comorbidities.
2. Involve family or major caregivers in treatment.
3. Assess and monitor frequently.
4. Consider behavioral, psychological, and social correlates of weight gain in treatment plan.
5. Recommend dietary changes and physical activity increases that can be implemented within family environment.
6. Recommend creation of "active school communities."[d]
7. Data supporting use of pharmacologic therapy for pediatric overweight are limited and inconclusive.
8. Adolescent candidates for bariatric surgery should have BMI ≥ 40, have attained a majority of skeletal maturity, and have obesity-related comorbidity. Refer to centers with experience in meeting unique needs of adolescents and that are collecting long-term outcomes data.

Footnotes:

[a]Children younger than 2 years should be referred to a pediatric obesity center.

[b]Evaluate for: 1. Exogenous causes: genetic syndromes, hypothyroidism, Cushing's syndrome, eating disorders, depression; 2. Complications: hypertension, dyslipidemias, noninsulin-dependent diabetes mellitus, slipped capital femoral epiphysis, pseudotumor cerebri, sleep apnea or obesity hypoventilation syndrome, gallbladder disease, polycystic ovary disease.

[c]Use change in BMI to identify rate of excessive weight gain relative to linear growth.

[d]RCT of weight management group participation (2x/week for 6 months, then every other week for 6 months; exercise and nutrition/behavior modification) among children aged 8–16 years: sustained (12-month) improvements in weight, BMI, body fat, and insulin resistance. (JAMA 2007;297:2697–2704)

Pediatrics 2006;117:1834–1842. Pediatrics 2003;112:424–430.
Circulation 2005;111:1999–2012. Pediatrics 2004;114:217–223.

OBESITY MANAGEMENT: CHILDREN
Treatment Recommendation: Children aged 2–9 years
with BMI > 85th percentile:
Source: **Expert Committee, Department of Health and Human Services**

Stage 1: Prevention Plus
(primary care with some training in pediatric weight management/ behavioral counseling)

Goal: Weight maintenance with growth. Proceed to Stage 2 if no improvement in 3–6 months.

Stage 2: Structured Weight Management
(primary care highly trained in weight management)

Goal: Weight maintenance with growth. Proceed to Stage 3 if no improvement in 3–6 months.

Stage 3: Comprehensive Multi-Disciplinary Protocol
(refer to multi-disciplinary obesity team)

Goal: Weight maintenance or gradual weight loss to BMI < 85th percentile. If BMI > 95th percentile with comorbidities, or no improvement with Stages 1–3, or BMI > 99th percentile, proceed to Stage 4.

Stage 4: Tertiary Care
(consideration of meal replacement, very-low-calorie diet, medication, surgery)

Source: http://ama-assn.org/ama1/pub/upload/mm/433/ped_obesity_recs.pdf

OSTEOPOROSIS: MANAGEMENT[c]
Source: American Association of Clinical Endocrinologists, 2003

Known osteoporotic low-trauma fracture or osteoporosis by DEXA[a]

Treatment for all:
+ Pharmacologic Management[b]

Treatment for all:
- Calcium supplementation 1,000–1,500 mg/day
- Vitamin D 400–800 IU/day
- Weight-bearing exercise 30 min/day, 3 days/week
- Strongly discourage tobacco
- Avoid glucocorticoids
- Hip protectors if high fall risk

Agents approved for treatment of osteoporosis:
- Bisphosphonates (alendronate, risedronate)
  - ↑ BMD of spine, hip and ↓ vertebral and nonvertebral fracture risk
- Calcitonin
  - ↓ vertebral but *not* nonvertebral fracture risk
  - Modest ↑ spinal BMD
  - Analgesic effect in acute osteoporotic fracture
- Estrogen
  - Must individualize risk/benefit assessment
  - ↓ vertebral and hip fracture risk
- Selective estrogen receptor modulators (SERMs—raloxifene)
  - Modest ↑ BMD spine and hip
  - ↓ vertebral fracture risk
  - No documented ↓ in nonvertebral fracture risk
- Parathyroid hormone (teriparatide)
  - Subcutaneous injection
  - ↓ risk of vertebral and nonvertebral fractures

[a]Indications for treatment
- ♀ with T scores below –2.5 in the absence of risk factors
- ♀ with T scores –1.5 to –2.5 if other risk factors present (see page 76)
- Prior vertebral or hip fracture

[b]Selection of pharmacologic agents for treating osteoporosis should be based on individual risk/benefit and preferences. Bisphosphonates are indicated for male osteoporosis and for glucocorticoid-induced osteoporosis. Alendronate: Has been shown to increase BMD by 5%–10% and to decrease fracture incidence by 50%. [Recommended dose: 5 mg/day (35 mg/week) for recently menopausal women; 10 mg/day (70 mg/week) for established osteoporosis. Treatment efficacy demonstrated for 7 years.] Risedronate: Has been shown to increase BMD and decrease fracture incidence by 30%–50%. (Recommended dose 5 mg/day or 35 mg/week.) Raloxifene: Has been shown to decrease the risk of vertebral fracture by 50% and to increase BMD. (Recommended dosing: 60 mg/day.)

OSTEOPOROSIS: MANAGEMENT[c] (CONTINUED)
Source: American Association of Clinical Endocrinologists

[c]Follow-up: perform follow-up BMD yearly for 2 years. If bone mass stabilizes after 2 years, remeasure every 2 years. Otherwise, continue annual BMD until bone mass is stable. Medicare covers BMD every 2 years. Biochemical markers of BME turnover can be used to monitor response to treatment.

Source: Adapted from AACE 2003 Medical Guidelines for Clinical Practice for the Prevention and Management of Postmenopausal Osteoporosis.

Evidence Updates
1. Fracture Intervention Trial: Alendronate decreased vertebral fracture risk (relative risk 0.57 for radiographic fracture) for women with T scores −1.6 to −2.5 (femoral neck). [Mayo Clin Proc 2005 Mar;80(3):343–9]
2. Alendronate therapy not cost effective for postmenopausal women with T scores better than −2.5 and no fracture history or other risk factors. [Ann Intern Med, 2005 May 3; 142(9):734–41]
3. Once yearly 15-minute intravenous zoledronic acid decreases vertebral (−70%) and hip (−40%) fracture risk over 3-year period. (NEJM 2007;356:1809)

PALLIATIVE AND END-OF-LIFE CARE: PAIN MANAGEMENT

PRINCIPLES OF ANALGESIC USE

By the mouth	The oral route is the preferred route for analgesics, including morphine.
By the clock	Persistent pain requires around-the-clock treatment to prevent further pain. PRN dosing is irrational and inhumane; it requires patients to experience pain before becoming eligible for relief.
By the WHO ladder	If a maximum dose of medication fails to adequately relieve pain, move up the ladder, not laterally to a different drug in the same efficiency group. Severe pain requires immediate use of an opioid recommended for controlling severe pain, without progressing sequentially through Steps 1 and 2.
Individualize treatment	The right dose of an analgesic is the dose that relieves pain with acceptable side effects for a specific patient.
Monitor	Monitoring is required to ensure the benefits of treatment are maximized while adverse effects are minimized.
Use adjuvant drugs	For example, an NSAID is almost always needed to help control bone pain. Nonopioid analgesics, such as NSAIDs or acetaminophen, can be used at any step of the ladder. Adjuvant medications also can be used at any step to enhance pain relief or counteract the adverse effects of medications.

Reprinted with permission from the American Academy of Hospice and Palliative Medicine. *Pocket Guide to Hospice/Palliative Medicine.*

PALLIATIVE AND END-OF-LIFE CARE: PAIN MANAGEMENT

WORLD HEALTH ORGANIZATION (WHO) ANALGESIC LADDER

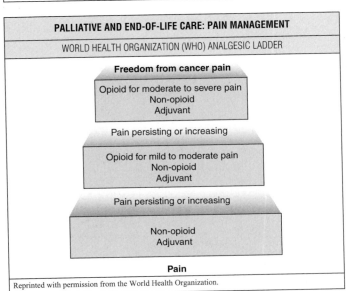

Freedom from cancer pain

Opioid for moderate to severe pain
Non-opioid
Adjuvant

Pain persisting or increasing

Opioid for mild to moderate pain
Non-opioid
Adjuvant

Pain persisting or increasing

Non-opioid
Adjuvant

Pain

Reprinted with permission from the World Health Organization.

PAP SMEAR ABNORMALITIES: MANAGEMENT AND FOLLOW-UP[a]
Source: Adapted from ICSI

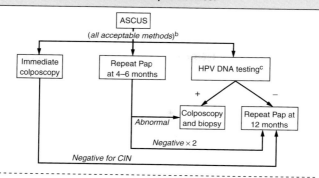

Cellular Abnormality	Recommended Follow-Up	Comments
Benign endometrial cells	Endometrial biopsy	Menopausal women only
Atypical glandular cells	Colposcopy and ECC	Endometrial biopsy if age ≥ 35, abnormal bleeding, morbid obesity, oligomenorrhea
ASC-H	Colposcopy	
LSIL	Colposcopy	
HSIL	Colposcopy with biopsy and/or LEEP	
Adenocarcinoma in situ, squamous cell carcinoma	Refer to gynecology or gynoncology	

[a] Assumes satisfactory specimen; if unsatisfactory, repeat Pap smear. If no endocervical cells, follow up in 1 year for low risk with previously negative smear, repeat in 4–6 mo for high risk.

[b] Post-menopausal women: provide a course of intravaginal estrogen followed by repeat Pap smear 1 week after completing therapy. If repeat Pap negative, repeat in 4–6 months. If negative × 2, return to routine screening. If repeat test ASCUS or greater, refer for colposcopy. Immunosuppressed women should have immediate referral to colposcopy.

[c] NCI, ASCCP, and ACS recommend that HPV testing may be added to routine PAP smear testing in women ≥ 30 years. Women with negative PAP and HPV can be rescreened every 3 years. (Obstet Gynecol 2004;103:304) Atypical squamous cells of undetermined significance/low-grade squamous intraepithelial lesion triage study (ALTS): Triage based on HPV DNA testing for women with ASCUS cytology is an economically viable option. (J Natl Cancer Inst 2006;98:92–100) Inverse relationship between age and HPV positivity for women with ASCUS. Given high prevalence of HPV and low occurrence of high-grade lesions in women aged ≤ 25 years with ASCUS, an HPV-based triage strategy will result in the referral of large numbers for colposcopy and may decrease the cost-effectiveness and clinical usefulness of this strategy. (Obstet Gynecol 2006;107:822–829) Women with HPV-negative ASCUS have very low absolute risk of subsequent CIN3 or worse in the subsequent 2 years. At 12-month follow-up visit, HPV testing has higher specificity and lower referrals than cytology. (Obstet Gynecol 2007;109:1325–1331)

PAP SMEAR ABNORMALITIES: MANAGEMENT AND FOLLOW-UP[a] (CONTINUED)

[d]Initial colposcopy may be deferred in adolescents with LSIL. May manage with repeat Pap at 6 and 12 months or HPV DNA testing at 12 months with referral to colposcopy for ASCUS or greater or high-risk HPV DNA types.

ASCUS = atypical squamous cells of undetermined significance; ECC = endocervical curettage; LSIL = low-grade squamous intraepithelial lesion; CIN = cervical intraepithelial neoplasia; HSIL = high-grade squamous intraepithelial lesion; CIS = carcinoma in situ ASC-H = atypical squamous cells, cannot exclude HSIL; LEEP = 100p electrosurgical excision

Source: Modified from JAMA 2002;287:2120–2129 and ICSI (http://www.icsi.org)

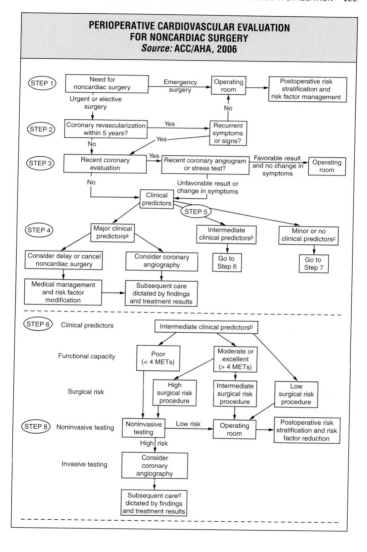

PERIOPERATIVE CARDIOVASCULAR EVALUATION FOR NONCARDIAC SURGERY
Source: ACC/AHA, 2006

PERIOPERATIVE CARDIOVASCULAR EVALUATION FOR NONCARDIAC SURGERY (CONTINUED)
Source: ACC/AHA, 2006

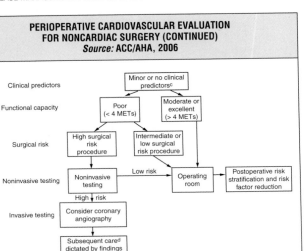

Footnotes:

[a]<u>Major Clinical Predictors</u>

- Unstable coronary syndromes
- Decompensated CHF
- Significant arrhythmias
- Severe valvular disease

[b]<u>Intermediate Clinical Predictors</u>

- Mild angina pectoris
- Prior MI
- Compensated or prior CHF
- Diabetes mellitus
- Renal insufficiency

[c]<u>Minor Clinical Predictors</u>

- Advanced age
- Abnormal ECG
- Rhythm other than sinus
- Low functional capacity
- History of stroke
- Uncontrolled systemic hypertension

[d]Subsequent care may include cancellation or delay of surgery, coronary revascularization followed by noncardiac surgery, or intensified care.

Perioperative beta-blocker therapy recommended for:
1. Patients undergoing surgery who are receiving beta-blockers for angina, symptomatic arrhythmias, or hypertension
2. Patients undergoing vascular surgery who are found to have myocardial ischemia or preoperative testing

Perioperative beta-blocker therapy probably recommended for:

Patients undergoing vascular, intermediate or high risk surgery in whom preoperative assessment identifies CHD or multiple cardiac risk factors

Source: Adapted from Eagle KA, Berger PB, Calkins H, et al. ACC/AHA guideline update for perioperative cardiovascular evaluation for noncardiac surgery update: a report of the American College of Cardiology/American Heart Association Task Force on Practice Guidelines (Committee to Update the 1996 Guidelines on Perioperative Cardiovascular Evaluation for Noncardiac Surgery). 2002. (http://www.acc.org, http://www.americanheart.org.downloadable/heart/perioperative.pdf) Update 2006 on Beta-Blocker Therapy Recommendations. JACC 2006;47:2343–2355.

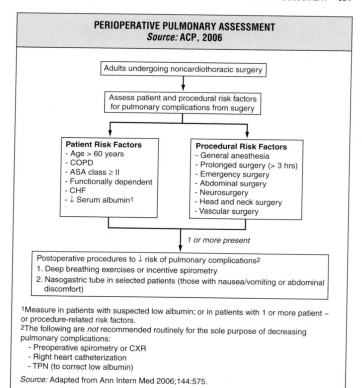

PERIOPERATIVE PULMONARY ASSESSMENT
Source: ACP, 2006

Adults undergoing noncardiothoracic surgery

Assess patient and procedural risk factors
for pulmonary complications from sugery

Patient Risk Factors
- Age > 60 years
- COPD
- ASA class ≥ II
- Functionally dependent
- CHF
- ↓ Serum albumin[1]

Procedural Risk Factors
- General anesthesia
- Prolonged surgery (> 3 hrs)
- Emergency surgery
- Abdominal surgery
- Neurosurgery
- Head and neck surgery
- Vascular surgery

1 or more present

Postoperative procedures to ↓ risk of pulmonary complications[2]
1. Deep breathing exercises or incentive spirometry
2. Nasogastric tube in selected patients (those with nausea/vomiting or abdominal discomfort)

[1]Measure in patients with suspected low albumin; or in patients with 1 or more patient – or procedure-related risk factors.
[2]The following are *not* recommended routinely for the sole purpose of decreasing pulmonary complications:
- Preoperative spirometry or CXR
- Right heart catheterization
- TPN (to correct low albumin)

Source: Adapted from Ann Intern Med 2006;144:575.

PNEUMONIA, COMMUNITY-ACQUIRED: EVALUATION
Source: IDSA, ATS, 2007

Diagnostic testing
- CXR or other chest imaging required for diagnosis
- Sputum gram stain and culture
  - Outpatients: optional
  - Inpatients: if unusual or antibiotic resistance suspected

Admission decision
- Severity of illness (eg, CURB-65) & prognostic indices (eg, PSI) support decision
- One must still recognize social and individual factors

CURB-65
(Thorax 2003;58:337–382)

Clinical factor	Points
Confusion	1
Blood urea nitrogen > 19 mg/dL	1
Respiratory rate ≥ 30 breaths/min	1
Systolic blood pressure < 90 mm Hg or Diastolic blood pressure ≤ 60 mm Hg	1
Age ≥ 65 years	1
Total points	

- CURB-65 ≥ 2 suggest need for hospitalization

Score	In-hospital mortality
0	0.7%
1	3.2%
2	3.0%
3	17%
4	42%
5	57%

Pneumonia Severity Index
(NEJM 1997;336:243–250)

	Points
Demographic factor	
Men age	age in years
Women age	age in years −10
Nursing home resident	+10
Co-existing illnesses	
Neoplastic disease	+30
Liver disease	+20
Congestive heart failure	+10
Cerebrovascular disease	+10
Renal disease	+10
Physical examination findings	
Altered mental status	+20
Respiratory rate 30 breaths/min	+20
Systolic BP < 90 mm Hg	+20
Temperature < 35°C (95°F)	+15
Temperature > 40°C (104°F)	+15
Pulse > 125 beats/min	+10
Laboratory and radiographic findings	
Arterial blood pH < 7.35	+30
BUN > 30 mg/dL	+20
Sodium level < 130 mmcl/L	+20
Glucose level > 250 mg/dL	+10
Hematocrit < 30%	+10
PaO_2 < 60 mmHg or O_2 sat. < 90%	+10
Pleural effusion	+10

Add up total points to estimate mortality risk

Class	Points	Overall Mortality
I	<51	0.1%
II	51–70	0.6%
III	71–90	0.9%
IV	91–130	9.5%
V	>130	26.7%

Source: IDSA and ATS Consensus Guidelines, 2007. (Clin Infect Diseases 2007;44:S27–72) Pneumonia Severity Index. (NEJM 1997;336:243)

PNEUMONIA, COMMUNITY-ACQUIRED: TREATMENT
Source: IDSA, ATS, 2007

GROUP I
Outpatient
No sig. PMHx[1]
No DRSP risk factors[6]

Macrolide
or
Doxycycline

GROUP II
Outpatient
With sig. PMHx[1]
or DRSP risk factors[6]

Beta-Lactam[5]
plus
Macrolide (or doxycycline)
or
Fluoroquinolone[4]
or
Amoxicillin[3]-clavulanate

GROUP III
Inpatients[2]
Not ICU
No sig. PMHx[1]
No DRSP risk factors[6]

Macrolide
or
Doxycycline

GROUP IV
ICU inpatients[2]
With sig. PMHx[1]
or DRSP risk factors[6]

IV Beta-Lactam[5]
plus
IV azithromycin or
Fluoroquinolone[4]

- If *Pseudomonas* a consideration: pipericillin/tazobactam; cefipime; imipenem or meropenem plus ciprofloxacin or levofloxacin; OR the beta-lactam plus aminoglycoside and azithromycin; OR the beta-lactam plus aminoglycoside and anti-pneumococcal fluoroquinolone.

- If CA-MRSA a consideration: add vancomycin or linezolid.

DRSP = drug-resistant *S. pneumoniae;* PMHx = past medical history; CA-MRSA = community-acquired methicillin-resistant *S. aureus*

Footnotes

1. Significant past medical history: chronic heart, lung, liver, or renal disease; diabetes melitus; alcoholism; malignancies; asplenia; immunosuppression

2. 1st dose of antibiotics in emergency department

3. High-dose amoxicillin: 1 gm po tid or 2 gm po bid

4. Anti-pneumococcal Fluoroquinolones: gemifloxacin, moxifloxacin, or levofloxicin (750 mg)

5. Cefotaxime, ceftriaxone, or ampicillin-sulbactam

6. DRSP risk factors: age < 2 years or > 65 years, beta-lactam therapy within the previous 3 months, alcoholism, medical comorbidities, immunosuppressive illness or therapy, and exposure to a child in a day care center

Source: IDSA and ATS Consensus Guidelines, 2007. (Clin Infect Diseases 2007;44:S27–72)

PNEUMONIA, COMMUNITY-ACQUIRED: SUSPECTED PATHOGENS
Source: IDSA, ATS, 2007

Condition and Risk Factors	Commonly Encountered Pathogens
Alcoholism	*S. pneumoniae*, oral anaerobes, *K. pneumoniae*, *Acinetobacter* species, *M. tuberculosis*
COPD and/or smoking	*H. influenzae*, *P. aeruginosa*, *Legionella* species, *S. pneumoniae*, *M. catarrhalis*, *C. pneumoniae*
Aspiration	Gram-negative enteric pathogens, oral anaerobes
Lung abscess	CA-MRSA, oral anaerobes, endemic fungal pneumonia, *M. tuberculosis*, atypical mycobacteria
Exposure to bat or bird droppings	*H. capsulatum*
Exposure to birds	*C. psittaci* (if poultry: avian influenza)
Exposure to rabbits	*F. tularensis*
Exposure to farm animals or parturient cats	*C. burnetii* (Q fever)
HIV infection (early)	*S. pneumoniae*, *H. influenzae*, *M. tuberculosis*
HIV infection (late)	The pathogens listed for early infection plus *P. jirovecii*, *Cryptococcus*, *Histoplasma*, *Aspergillus*, atypical mycobacteria (especially *M. kansasii*), *P. aeruginosa*, *H. influenzae*
Hotel or cruise ship stay in previous 2 weeks	*Legionella* species
Travel to or residence in southwestern United States	*Coccidioides* species, *Hantavirus*
Travel to or residence in Southeast and East Asia	*B. pseudomallei*, avian influenza, SARS
Influenza active in community	Influenza, *S. pneumoniae*, *S. aureus*, *H. influenzae*
Cough ≥ 2 weeks with whoop or posttussive vomiting	*B. pertussis*
Structural lung disease (eg, bronchiectasis)	*P. aeruginosa*, *B. cepacia*, *S. aureus*
Injection drug use	*S. aureus*, anaerobes, *M. tuberculosis*, *S. pneumoniae*
Endobronchial obstruction	Anaerobes, *S. pneumoniae*, *H. influenzae*, *S. aureus*
In context of bioterrorism	*B. anthracis* (anthrax), *Y. pestis* (plague), *F. tularensis* (tularemia)

CA-MRSA = community-acquired methicillin-resistant *Staphylococcus aureus*; COPD = chronic obstructive pulmonary disease; SARS = severe acute respiratory syndrome

ROUTINE PRENATAL CARE
Source: ICSI, 2006

Event[1]	Preconception Visit[2]	Visit 1[3]** (6–8 Weeks)	Visit 2 (10–12 Weeks)	Visit 3 (16–18 Weeks)	Visit 4 (22 Weeks)
Screening maneuvers	Risk profiles[4] Height and weight/BMI[5] Blood pressure[6] History and physical[7] Cholesterol and HDL[2] Cervical cancer screening[3] Rubella/rubeola[8] Varicella[9] Domestic abuse[10]	Risk profiles[4] GC/*Chlamydia*[4] Height and weight/BMI[5] Blood pressure[6] History and physical[7]* Rubella[8] Varicella[9] Domestic abuse[10] Hemoglobin[15] ABO/Rh/Ab[16] Syphilis[17] Urine culture[18] HIV[19] [Blood lead screening[20]] [VBAC[21]] Hepatitis B S Ag[25]	Weight[5] Blood pressure[6] Fetal heart tones[27] Fetal anomaly/biochemical screening[23]	Weight[5] Blood pressure[6] Fetal heart tones[27] Fetal anomaly/biochemical screening[23] OB ultrasound (optional)[28] Fundal height[29] [Cervical assessment[30]]	Weight[5] Blood pressure[6] Fetal heart tones[27] Fundal height[29] [Cervical assessment[30]]

ROUTINE PRENATAL CARE (CONTINUED)
Source: ICSI, 2006

Event[1]	Preconception Visit[2]	Visit 1[3]** (6–8 Weeks)	Visit 2 (10–12 Weeks)	Visit 3 (16–18 Weeks)	Visit 4 (22 Weeks)
Counseling education intervention	PTL education and prevention[11] Substance use[2] Nutrition and weight[2] Domestic abuse[10] List of medications, herbal supplements, vitamins[12] Accurate recording of menstrual dates[13]	PTL education and prevention[11] Prenatal and lifestyle education[22] •Physical activity •Nutrition •Warning signs •Course of care •Physiology of pregnancy •Follow up modifiable risk factors Discuss fetal aneuploidy screening[23]	PTL education and prevention[11] Prenatal and lifestyle education[22] •Fetal growth •Review labs from visit 1 •Breastfeeding •Physiology of pregnancy •Follow up modifiable risk factors	PTL education and prevention[11] Prenatal and lifestyle education[22] •Physiology of pregnancy •Second trimester growth •Quickening •Follow up modifiable risk factors	PTL education and prevention[11] Prenatal and lifestyle education[22] •Classes •Family issues •Length of stay •Gestational diabetes mellitus[32] •Follow up modifiable risk factors •[RhoGam[16]]
Immunization and chemoprophylaxis	Tetanus booster[3] Rubella/MMR[4] [Varicella/VZIG[9]] Hepatitis B vaccine[7,25] Folic acid supplement[14]	Tetanus booster[3] Nutritional supplements[24] Influenza[26] [Varicella/VZIG[9]]		[Progesterone[31]]	

Superscript numbers refer to specific annotations (see http://www.icsi.org).
[Bracketed] items refer to high-risk groups only.
* It is acceptable for the history and physical laboratory tests listed under Visit 1 to be deferred to Visit 2 with the agreement of both the patient and the provider.
** Should also include all subjects listed for the preconception visit if none occurred.
PTL = preterm labor
Source: Copyright ©2006 by Institute for Clinical Systems Improvement. ICSI retains all rights to the material.

ROUTINE PRENATAL CARE (CONTINUED)
Source: ICSI, 2006

Event	Visit 5 (28 Weeks)	Visit 6 (32 Weeks)	Visit 7 (36 Weeks)	Visits 8–11 (38–41 Weeks)
Screening maneuvers	PTL risk[4] Weight[5] Blood pressure[6] Fetal heart tones[27] Fundal height[29] [Cervical assessment[30]] Gestational diabetes mellitus[32] Domestic abuse[10] [Rh antibody status[16]] [Hepatitis B Ag[25]] [GC/*Chlamydia*[4]]	Weight[5] Blood pressure[6] Fetal heart tones[27] Fundal height[29]	Weight[5] Blood pressure[6] Fetal heart tones[27] Fundal height[29] Cervix exam[34] Confirm fetal position[35] Culture for group B streptococcus[36]	Weight[5] Blood pressure[6] Fetal heart tones[27] Fundal height[29] Cervix exam[34]

ROUTINE PRENATAL CARE (CONTINUED)
Source: ICSI, 2006

Event	Visit 5 (28 Weeks)	Visit 6 (32 Weeks)	Visit 7 (36 Weeks)	Visits 8–11 (38–41 Weeks)		
Counseling education intervention	PTL labor education and prevention[11] Prenatal and lifestyle education[22] •Work •Physiology of pregnancy •Preregistration •Fetal growth •Follow up modifiable risk factors Awareness of fetal movement[33]	PTL labor education and prevention[11] Prenatal and lifestyle education[22] •Travel •Sexuality •Pediatric care •Episiotomy •Follow up modifiable risk factors Labor and delivery issues Warning signs/PIH [VBAC[21]]	Prenatal and lifestyle education[22] •Postpartum care •Management of late pregnancy symptoms •Contraception •When to call provider •Discussion of postpartum depression •Follow up modifiable risk factors	Prenatal and lifestyle education[22] •Postpartum vaccinations •Infant CPR •Post-term management •Follow up modifiable risk factors Labor and delivery update		
Immunization and chemoprophylaxis	[ABO/Rh/Ab[16]] [RhoGAM[16]]					

Superscript numbers refer to specific annotations (see http://www.icsi.org).

[Bracketed] items refer to high-risk groups only.

PTL = preterm labor; PIH = pregnancy-induced hypertension

Source: Copyright ©2006 by Institute for Clinical Systems Improvement. ICSI retains all rights to the material.

PERI- AND POSTNATAL GUIDELINES *Source:* AAP, AAFP	
Breastfeeding	Strongly recommends education and counseling to promote breastfeeding.
Hemoglobinopathies	Strongly recommends ordering screening tests for hemoglobinopathies in neonates.
Hyperbilirubinemia	Perform ongoing systematic assessments during the neonatal period for the risk of an infant developing severe hyperbilirubinemia.
Phenylketonuria	Strongly recommends ordering screening tests for phenylketonuria in neonates.
Thyroid function abnormalities	Strongly recommends ordering screening tests for thyroid function abnormalities in neonates.

Source: Pediatrics 2004;114:297–316; Pediatrics 2005;115:496–506. (http://www.aafp.org/online/en/home/clinical/exam.html)

TOBACCO CESSATION TREATMENT ALGORITHM
Source: U.S. Public Health Service

Five A's
1. Ask about tobacco use.
2. Advise to quit through clear personalized messages.
3. Assess willingness to quit.
4. Assist to quit,[a] including referral to Quit Lines (eg, 1-800-NO-BUTTS).
5. Arrange follow-up and support.

[a]Physicians can assist patients to quit by devising a quit plan, providing problem-solving counseling, providing intratreatment social support, helping patients obtain social support from their environment/friends, and recommending pharmacotherapy for appropriate patients. Use caution in recommending pharmacotherapy in patients with medical contraindications, those smoking < 10 cigarettes per day, pregnant/breastfeeding women, and adolescent smokers. As of March 2005, Medicare covers costs for smoking cessation counseling for those who (1) have a smoking-related illness; (2) have an illness complicated by smoking; or (3) take a medication that is made less effective by smoking. (http://www.cms.hhs.gov/mcd/viewdecisionmemo.asp?id=130)
Source: Fiore MC et al. Treating Tobacco Use and Dependence. Quick Reference Guide for Clinicians. Rockville, MD: U.S. Department of Health and Human Services. Public Health Service, October 2000.

MOTIVATING TOBACCO USERS TO QUIT

Five R's
1. Relevance: personal
2. Risks: acute, long-term, environmental
3. Rewards: have patient identify (eg, save money, better food taste)
4. Road blocks: help problem-solve
5. Repetition: at every office visit

TOBACCO CESSATION TREATMENT OPTIONS[a]

First-line pharmacotherapies (approved for use for smoking cessation by the FDA)

Pharmacotherapy	Precautions/ Contraindications	Side Effects	Dosage	Duration	Availability	Cost/Day[b]
Bupropion SR	History of seizure History of eating disorder	Insomnia Dry mouth	150 mg every morning for 3 days, then 150 mg twice daily. (Begin treatment 1–2 weeks pre-quit.)	7–12 weeks maintenance up to 6 months	Zyban (prescription only)	$5.73
Nicotine gum	—	Mouth soreness Dyspepsia	1–24 cigs/day: 2-mg gum (up to 24 pieces/day). 25+ cigs/day: 4-mg gum (up to 24 pieces/day).	Up to 12 weeks	Nicorette, Nicorette Mint (OTC only)	$5.81
Nicotine inhaler	—	Local irritation of mouth and throat	6–16 cartridges/day	Up to 6 months	Nicotrol Inhaler (prescription only)	$6.07
Nicotine nasal spray	—	Nasal irritation	8–40 doses/day	3–6 months	Nicotrol NS (prescription only)	$3.67
Nicotine patch	—	Local skin reaction Insomnia	21 mg/24 hours 14 mg/24 hours 7 mg/24 hours 15 mg/16 hours	4 weeks Then 2 weeks Then 2 weeks 8 weeks	Nicoderm CQ (OTC only), generic patches (prescription and OTC) Nicotrol (OTC only)	$3.91
Varenicline	Renal impairment	Nausea Abnormal dreams	0.5 mg QD for 3 days, then 0.5 mg twice daily for 4 days, then 1.0 mg po twice daily	12 weeks or 24 weeks	Chantix (prescription only)	$4.22

TOBACCO CESSATION TREATMENT OPTIONS

TOBACCO CESSATION TREATMENT OPTIONS[a] (CONTINUED)

Pharmacotherapy	Precautions/ Contraindications	Side Effects	Dosage	Duration	Availability	Cost/Day[c]
Second-line pharmacotherapies (not approved for use for smoking cessation by the FDA)						
Clonidine	Rebound hypertension	Dry mouth Drowsiness Dizziness Sedation	0.15–0.75 mg/day	3–10 weeks	Oral Clonidine-generic, Catapres (prescription only), Transdermal Catapres (prescription only)	Clonidine $0.24 for 0.2 mg; Catapres (transdermal) $3.50
Nortriptyline	Risk of arrhythmias	Sedation Dry mouth	75–100 mg/day	12 weeks	Nortriptyline HCl-generic (prescription only)	$0.74 for 75 mg

[a]The information contained within this table is not comprehensive. Please see package insert for additional information.
[b]Prices from Rx for Change, the Regents of the University of California, University of Southern California, and Western University of Health Sciences.
[c]Prices based on retail prices of a national chain pharmacy; 2000.
Source: U.S. Public Health Service.

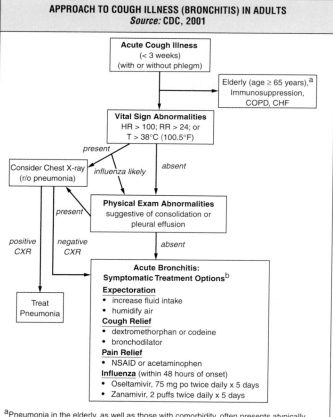

APPROACH TO COUGH ILLNESS (BRONCHITIS) IN ADULTS
Source: CDC, 2001

Acute Cough Illness
(< 3 weeks)
(with or without phlegm)

Elderly (age ≥ 65 years),[a]
Immunosuppression,
COPD, CHF

Vital Sign Abnormalities
HR > 100; RR > 24; or
T > 38°C (100.5°F)

present → Consider Chest X-ray (r/o pneumonia)

influenza likely

absent

Physical Exam Abnormalities
suggestive of consolidation or
pleural effusion

present

positive CXR / *negative CXR*

absent

Treat Pneumonia

Acute Bronchitis:
Symptomatic Treatment Options[b]

Expectoration
- increase fluid intake
- humidify air

Cough Relief
- dextromethorphan or codeine
- bronchodilator

Pain Relief
- NSAID or acetaminophen

Influenza (within 48 hours of onset)
- Oseltamivir, 75 mg po twice daily x 5 days
- Zanamivir, 2 puffs twice daily x 5 days

[a] Pneumonia in the elderly, as well as those with comorbidity, often presents atypically. Evaluation should be individualized.

[b] If duration of illness is > 2 weeks, consider pertusis. PCR or culture testing for pertussis is done to confirm the diagnosis and indicate the need for public health follow-up to prevent illness among contacts, especially infants. Antibiotic therapy can decrease shedding, but has no effect on symptoms during the paroxysmal phase (≥ 10 days after illness onset). Treat with erythromycin x 14 days pending results.

Source: Adapted from Centers for Disease Control and Prevention; Ann Intern Med 2001; 134:521.

APPROACH TO ACUTE SORE THROAT (PHARYNGITIS) IN ADULTS
Source: CDC, 2001

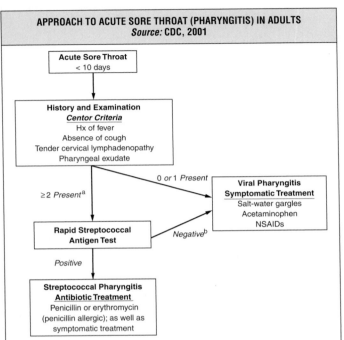

Acute Sore Throat
< 10 days

History and Examination
Centor Criteria
Hx of fever
Absence of cough
Tender cervical lymphadenopathy
Pharyngeal exudate

0 or 1 Present → **Viral Pharyngitis**
Symptomatic Treatment
Salt-water gargles
Acetaminophen
NSAIDs

≥2 Present[a]

Rapid Streptococcal Antigen Test

Negative[b]

Positive

Streptococcal Pharyngitis
Antibiotic Treatment
Penicillin or erythromycin
(penicillin allergic); as well as
symptomatic treatment

[a]Acceptable alternatives to these strategies include: 1) test and treat patients with 2 or 3 Centor criteria present, and empirically treat with antibiotics (do not test) patients with 4 Centor criteria; or 2) do not test any patients, and empirically treat with antibiotics patients with 3 or 4 Centor criteria present.

[b]Do not recommend culture-confirmation of negative rapid antigen tests in adults when the sensitivity of the rapid antigen test exceeds 80%. When performed in adults with ≥ 2 criteria present, the sensitivity exceeds 90%. (Ann Emerg Med 2001;38:648)

These principles apply to immunocompetent adults without complicated comorbidities such as chronic lung or heart disease, history of rheumatic fever, or during known group A streptococcal outbreaks. They also are not intended to apply during a known epidemic of acute rheumatic fever or streptococcal pharyngitis, or for nonindustrialized countries where the endemic rate of acute rheumatic fever is much higher than it is in the U.S.

Source: Adapted from Centers for Disease Control and Prevention; Ann Intern Med 2001; 134:509.

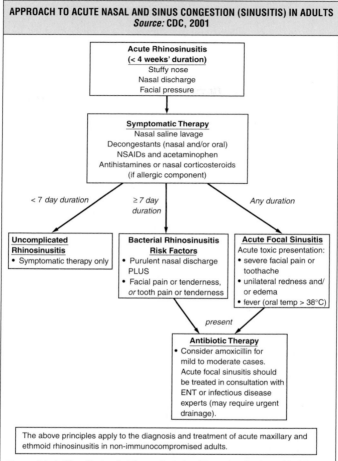

APPROACH TO ACUTE NASAL AND SINUS CONGESTION (SINUSITIS) IN ADULTS
Source: **CDC, 2001**

**Acute Rhinosinusitis
(< 4 weeks' duration)**
Stuffy nose
Nasal discharge
Facial pressure

↓

Symptomatic Therapy
Nasal saline lavage
Decongestants (nasal and/or oral)
NSAIDs and acetaminophen
Antihistamines or nasal corticosteroids
(if allergic component)

< 7 day duration   *≥ 7 day duration*   *Any duration*

Uncomplicated Rhinosinusitis
• Symptomatic therapy only

Bacterial Rhinosinusitis Risk Factors
• Purulent nasal discharge PLUS
• Facial pain or tenderness, *or* tooth pain or tenderness

Acute Focal Sinusitis
Acute toxic presentation:
• severe facial pain or toothache
• unilateral redness and/ or edema
• fever (oral temp > 38°C)

present

Antibiotic Therapy
• Consider amoxicillin for mild to moderate cases. Acute focal sinusitis should be treated in consultation with ENT or infectious disease experts (may require urgent drainage).

The above principles apply to the diagnosis and treatment of acute maxillary and ethmoid rhinosinusitis in non-immunocompromised adults.

Source: Adapted from Centers for Disease Control and Prevention; Ann Intern Med 2001; 134:498

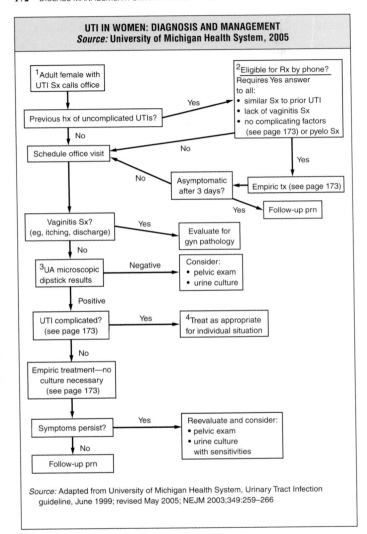

UTI IN WOMEN: DIAGNOSIS AND MANAGEMENT
Source: **University of Michigan Health System, 2005**

Source: Adapted from University of Michigan Health System, Urinary Tract Infection guideline, June 1999; revised May 2005; NEJM 2003;349:259–266

UTI IN WOMEN ALGORITHM, NOTES AND TABLES

LABORATORY CHARGES AND RELATIVE COSTS

Test	Relative Cost
Urinalysis, dipstick	$
Urinalysis, complete microscopic	$$
Urine culture	$$$

COMPLICATING FACTORS

Catheter
Diabetes mellitus
Immunosuppression
Nephrolithiasis present
Pregnancy
Pyelonephritis symptoms (fever, nausea, back pain)
Recent hospitalization or nursing home residence
Recurrent UTIs (3/year)
Symptoms for > 7 days
Urologic structural/functional abnormality

TREATMENT REGIMENS AND RELATIVE COSTS

Treatment Regimen	Relative Cost (generic)
First Line	
Trimethoprim/Sulfa DS BID × 3 days	$
Second Line (in preferred order)	
Ciprofloxacin 250 mg BID × 3 days	$
Levofloxacin 250 mg QID × 3 days	$$$$
Amoxicillin 500 mg TID × 7 days	$$
Nitrofurantoin 100 mg QID × 7 days	$$
Macrobid 100 mg BID × 7 days	$$

1. The majority of UTIs occur in sexually active women. Risk increases by 3–5 times when diaphragms are used for contraception. Risk also increases slightly with not voiding after sexual intercourse and use of spermicides. Dysuria with either urgency or frequency, in the absence of vaginal symptoms, yields a prior probability of UTI of 70%–80%. Generally, UTI symptoms are of abrupt onset (< 3 days).
2. Guideline implementation decreases the proportion of patients with presumed cystitis who received urinalysis, urine culture, or an initial office visit and increases the proportion of women who receive a guideline-recommended antibiotic. Adverse outcomes (return office visit, sexually transmitted disease, pyelonephritis within 60 days of initial diagnosis) did not increase as a result of guideline implementation. (Saint S, et al. Am J Med 1999;106:636–641)
3. *Dipstick analysis* for leukocyte esterase, an indirect test for the presence for pyuria, is the least expensive and least time-intensive diagnostic test for UTI. It is estimated to have a sensitivity of 75%–96% and specificity of 94%–98%. Nitrite testing by dipstick is less useful, in large part because it is only positive in the presence of bacteria that produce nitrate reductase, and can be confounded by consumption of ascorbic acid. *Microscopic examination* of unstained, centrifuged urine by a trained observer under 40× power has a sensitivity of 82%–97% and a specificity of 84%–95%. For urine culture, sensitivity varies from 50%–95%, depending on the threshold for UTI, and specificity varies from 85%–99%. Because of the limited sensitivity of urine culture, and the delay required for results, urine culture is not recommended to diagnose or verify uncomplicated UTI.
4. Unlike women with uncomplicated UTI, care for women with complicating factors includes:
   • *Culture:* Obtain pretreatment culture and sensitivity.
   • *Treatment:* Initiate treatment with trimethoprim/sulfa or quinolone for 7–14 days (quinolones contraindicated in pregnancy).
   • *Follow-up UA:* Obtain follow-up urinalysis to document clearing.
   • *Possible structural evaluation:* Lower threshold for urologic structural evaluation with cysto/IVP.

4
Appendices

SCREENING INSTRUMENTS: ALCOHOL ABUSE

SENSITIVITY AND SPECIFICITY OF SCREENING TESTS FOR PROBLEM DRINKING

Instrument Name	Screening Questions/Scoring	Threshold Score	Sensitivity/Specificity (%)	Source
CAGE[a]	See page 177	> 1 > 2 > 3	77/58 53/81 29/92	Am J Psychiatry 1974;131:1121 J Gen Intern Med 1998;13:379
AUDIT	See page 177–178	> 4 > 5 > 6	87/70 77/84 66/90	BMJ 1997;314:420 J Gen Intern Med 1998;13:379

[a]The CAGE may be less applicable to binge drinkers (eg, college students), the elderly, and minority populations.

SCREENING INSTRUMENTS: ALCOHOL ABUSE

SCREENING PROCEDURES FOR PROBLEM DRINKING

1. CAGE screening test[a]

Have you ever felt the need to	**C**ut down on drinking?
Have you ever felt	**A**nnoyed by criticism of your drinking?
Have you ever felt	**G**uilty about your drinking?
Have you ever taken a morning	**E**ye opener?

INTERPRETATION: Two "yes" answers are considered a positive screen. One "yes" answer should arouse a suspicion of alcohol abuse.

2. The Alcohol Use Disorder Identification Test (AUDIT).[b] (Scores for response categories are given in parentheses. Scores range from 0 to 40, with a cutoff score of ≥ 5 indicating hazardous drinking, harmful drinking, or alcohol dependence.)

1) How often do you have a drink containing alcohol?

(0) Never	(1) Monthly or less	(2) Two to four times a month	(3) Two or three times a week	(4) Four or more times a week

2) How many drinks containing alcohol do you have on a typical day when you are drinking?

(0) 1 or 2	(1) 3 or 4	(2) 5 or 6	(3) 7 to 9	(4) 10 or more

3) How often do you have six or more drinks on one occasion?

(0) Never	(1) Less than monthly	(2) Monthly	(3) Weekly	(4) Daily or almost daily

4) How often during the past year have you found that you were not able to stop drinking once you had started?

(0) Never	(1) Less than monthly	(2) Monthly	(3) Weekly	(4) Daily or almost daily

5) How often during the past year have you failed to do what was normally expected of you because of drinking?

(0) Never	(1) Less than monthly	(2) Monthly	(3) Weekly	(4) Daily or almost daily

SCREENING INSTRUMENTS: ALCOHOL ABUSE

SCREENING PROCEDURES FOR PROBLEM DRINKING (CONTINUED)

6) How often during the past year have you needed a first drink in the morning to get yourself going after a heavy drinking session?

(0) Never   (1) Less than monthly   (2) Monthly   (3) Weekly   (4) Daily or almost daily

7) How often during the past year have you had a feeling of guilt or remorse after drinking?

(0) Never   (1) Less than monthly   (2) Monthly   (3) Weekly   (4) Daily or almost daily

8) How often during the past year have you been unable to remember what happened the night before because you had been drinking?

(0) Never   (1) Less than monthly   (2) Monthly   (3) Weekly   (4) Daily or almost daily

9) Have you or has someone else been injured as a result of your drinking?

(0) No   (2) Yes, but not in the past year   (4) Yes, during the past year

10) Has a relative or friend or a doctor or other health worker been concerned about your drinking or suggested you cut down?

(0) No   (2) Yes, but not in the past year   (4) Yes, during the past year

[a]Modified from Mayfield D et al. The CAGE questionnaire: Validation of a new alcoholism screening instrument. Am J Psychiatry 1974;131:1121.
[b]From Piccinelli M et al. Efficacy of the alcohol use disorders identification test as a screening tool for hazardous alcohol intake and related disorders in primary care: A validity study. BMJ 1997;314:420.

SCREENING INSTRUMENTS:
COGNITIVE IMPAIRMENT

THE ANNOTATED MINI MENTAL STATE EXAMINATION (AMMSE)

MiniMental LLC

| Suspect dementia when score ≤ 24. |

NAME OF SUBJECT _____ Age _____

NAME OF EXAMINER _____ Years of School Completed ____

Approach the patient with respect and encouragement. Date of Examination _____

Ask: Do you have any trouble with your memory? ☐ Yes ☐ No

May I ask you some questions about your memory? ☐ Yes ☐ No

SCORE	ITEM

5 ( ) **TIME ORIENTATION**

Ask:

What is the year _____ (1), season _____ (1),

month of the year _____ (1), date _____ (1),

day of the week _____ (1)?

5 ( ) **PLACE ORIENTATION**

Ask:

Where are we now? What is the state _____ (1), city _____ (1),

part of the city _____ (1), building _____ (1),

floor of the building _____ (1)?

3 ( ) **REGISTRATION OF THREE WORDS**

Say: Listen carefully. I am going to say three words. You say them back after I stop. Ready? Here they are...PONY (wait 1 second), QUARTER (wait 1 second), ORANGE (wait 1 second). What were those words?

_____ (1)

_____ (1)

_____ (1)

Give 1 point for each correct answer, then repeat them until the patient learns all three.

5 ( ) **SERIAL 7s AS A TEST OF ATTENTION AND CALCULATION**

Ask: Subtract 7 from 100 and continue to subtract 7 from each subsequent remainder until I tell you to stop. What is 100 take away 7? _____ (1)

Say:

Keep going. _____ (1), _____ (1),

_____ (1), _____ (1),

3 ( ) **RECALL OF THREE WORDS**

Ask:

What were those three words I asked you to remember?

Give one point for each correct answer. _____ (1),

_____ (1), _____ (1),

2 ( ) **NAMING**

Ask:

What is this? (show pencil) _____ (1). What is this? (show watch) _____ (1).

For more information or additional copies of this exam, call (617)587-4215

© 1975, 1998 MiniMental LLC

SCREENING INSTRUMENTS:
COGNITIVE IMPAIRMENT (CONTINUED)

MiniMental LLC

1 ( )   **REPETITION**
Say:
Now I am going to ask you to repeat what I say. Ready? No ifs, ands or buts.
Now you say that. _____ (1)

3 ( )   **COMPREHENSION**
Say:
Listen carefully because I am going to ask you to do something.
Take this paper in your left hand (1), fold it in half (1), and put it on the floor. (1)

1 ( )   **READING**
Say:
Please read the following and do what it says, but do not say it aloud. (1)

Close your eyes

1 ( )   **WRITING**
Say:
Please write a sentence. If the patient does not respond, say: Write about the weather. (1)

_____
_____

1 ( )   **DRAWING**
Say: Please copy this design.

TOTAL SCORE _____   Assess level of consciousness along a continuum

Alert	Drowsy	Stupor	Coma

	YES NO			YES NO	FUNCTION BY PROXY

Cooperative: ☐ ☐   Deterioration from
Depressed: ☐ ☐   previous level of
Anxious: ☐ ☐   functioning: ☐ ☐
Poor Vision: ☐ ☐   Family History of Dementia: ☐ ☐
Poor Hearing: ☐ ☐   Head Trauma: ☐ ☐
Native Language: _____   Stroke: ☐ ☐
Alcohol Abuse: ☐ ☐
Thyroid Disease: ☐ ☐

FUNCTION BY PROXY
Please record date when patient was last
able to perform the following tasks.
Ask caregiver if patient independently handles:

	YES	NO	DATE
Money/Bills:	☐	☐	____
Medication:	☐	☐	____
Transportation:	☐	☐	____
Telephone:	☐	☐	____

Source: Reproduced with permission from "Mini-Mental State." A practical method for grading the cognitive state of patients for the clinician. J Psychiatr Res 1975;12(3):189. ©1975, 1998 MiniMental LLC.

SCREENING INSTRUMENTS: DEPRESSION

SCREENING TESTS FOR DEPRESSION

Instrument Name	Screening Questions/Scoring	Threshold Score	Source
Beck Depression Inventory (Short Form)	See page 184	0–4: None or minimal depression 5–7: Mild depression 8–15: Moderate depression > 15: Severe depression	Postgrad Med 1972;Dec:81
Geriatric Depression Scale	See page 185	≥ 15: Depression	J Psychiatr Res 1983;17:37
PRIME-MD© (mood questions)	(1) During the past month, have you often been bothered by feeling down, depressed, or hopeless? (2) During the past month, have you often been bothered by little interest or pleasure in doing things?	"Yes" to either question[a]	JAMA 1994;272:1749 J Gen Intern Med 1997;12:439
Patient Health Questionnaire (PHQ-9)©	http://www.pfizer.com/phq-9/ See page 182	*Major depressive syndrome:* if answers to #1a or b and ≥ 5 of #1a–i are at least "More than half the days" (count #1i if present at all). *Other depressive syndrome:* if #1a or b and 2–4 of #1a–i are at least "More than half the days" (count #1i if present at all). 5–9: mild depression 10–14: moderate depression 15–19: moderately severe depression 20–27: severe depression	JAMA 1999;282:1737 J Gen Intern Med 2001;16:606

[a]Sensitivity 86%–96%; specificity 57%–75%.
©Pfizer Inc.

SCREENING INSTRUMENTS: DEPRESSION (CONTINUED)

PHQ-9 DEPRESSION SCREEN, ENGLISH

**Over the <u>last 2 weeks</u>, how often have you been bothered
by any of the following problems?**

	Not at all	Several days	> Half the days	Nearly every day
a. Little interest or pleasure in doing things	0	1	2	3
b. Feeling down, depressed, or hopeless	0	1	2	3
c. Trouble falling or staying asleep, or sleeping too much	0	1	2	3
d. Feeling tired or having little energy	0	1	2	3
e. Poor appetite or overeating	0	1	2	3
f. Feeling bad about yourself—or that you are a failure or that you have let yourself or your family down	0	1	2	3
g. Trouble concentrating on things, such as reading the newspaper or watching television	0	1	2	3
h. Moving or speaking so slowly that other people could have noticed? Or the opposite—being so fidgety or restless that you have been moving around a lot more than usual	0	1	2	3
i. Thoughts that you would be better off dead or of hurting yourself in some way	0	1	2	3

(For office coding: Total Score ____ = ____ + ____ + ____ *)*

Major depressive syndrome: if ≥ 5 items present scored ≥ 2, and one of items is depressed mood (b) or anhedonia (a). If item "i" is present, then this counts, even if score = 1.
Depressive screen positive: if at least one item ≥ 2 (or item "i" is ≥ 1).

SCREENING INSTRUMENTS: DEPRESSION (CONTINUED)

PHQ-9 DEPRESSION SCREEN, SPANISH

Durante las <u>últimas 2 semanas</u>, ¿con qué frecuencia le han molestado los siguientes problemas?

	Nunca	Varios dias	> La mitad de los dias	Casi todos los dias
a. Tener poco interés o placer en hacer las cosas	0	1	2	3
b. Sentirse desanimada, deprimida, o sin esperanza	0	1	2	3
c. Con problemas en dormirse o en mantenerse dormida, o en dormir demasiado	0	1	2	3
d. Sentirse cansada o tener poca energía	0	1	2	3
e. Tener poco apetito o comer en exceso	0	1	2	3
f. Sentir falta de amor propio—o qe sea un fracaso o que decepcionara a sí misma o a su familia	0	1	2	3
g. Tener dificultad para concentrarse en cosas tales como leer el periódico o mirar la televisión	0	1	2	3
h. Se mueve o habla tan lentamente que otra gente se podría dar cuenta—o de lo contrario, está tan agitada o inquieta que se mueve mucho más de lo acostumbrado	0	1	2	3
i. Se le han ocurrido pensamientos de que se haría daño de alguna manera	0	1	2	3

(For office coding: Total Score _____ = _____ + _____ + _____)

SCREENING INSTRUMENTS: DEPRESSION

BECK DEPRESSION INVENTORY, SHORT FORM

Instructions: This is a questionnaire. On the questionnaire are groups of statements. Please read the entire group of statements in each category. Then pick out the one statement in that group that best describes the way you feel today, that is, *right now!* Circle the number beside the statement you have chosen. If several statements in the group seem to apply equally well, circle each one. Sum all numbers to calculate a score.

Be sure to read all the statements in each group before making your choice.

A. Sadness
3 I am so sad or unhappy that I can't stand it.
2 I am blue or sad all the time and I can't snap out of it.
1 I feel sad or blue.
0 I do not feel sad.

B. Pessimism
3 I feel that the future is hopeless and that things cannot improve.
2 I feel I have nothing to look forward to.
1 I feel discouraged about the future.
0 I am not particularly pessimistic or discouraged about the future.

C. Sense of failure
3 I feel I am a complete failure as a person (parent, husband, wife).
2 As I look back on my life, all I can see is a lot of failures.
1 I feel I have failed more than the average person.
0 I do not feel like a failure.

D. Dissatisfaction
3 I am dissatisfied with everything.
2 I don't get satisfaction out of anything anymore.
1 I don't enjoy things the way I used to.
0 I am not particularly dissatisfied.

E. Guilt
3 I feel as though I am very bad or worthless.
2 I feel quite guilty.
1 I feel bad or unworthy a good part of the time.
0 I don't feel particularly guilty.

F. Self-dislike
3 I hate myself.
2 I am disgusted with myself.
1 I am disappointed in myself.
0 I don't feel disappointed in myself.

G. Self-harm
3 I would kill myself if I had the chance.
2 I have definite plans about committing suicide.
1 I feel I would be better off dead.
0 I don't have any thoughts of harming myself.

H. Social withdrawal
3 I have lost all of my interest in other people and don't care about them at all.
2 I have lost most of my interest in other people and have little feeling for them.
1 I am less interested in other people than I used to be.
0 I have not lost interest in other people.

I. Indecisiveness
3 I can't make any decisions at all anymore.
2 I have great difficulty in making decisions.
1 I try to put off making decisions.
0 I make decisions about as well as ever.

J. Self-image change
3 I feel that I am ugly or repulsive-looking.
2 I feel that there are permanent changes in my appearance and they make me look unattractive.
1 I am worried that I am looking old or unattractive.
0 I don't feel that I look any worse than I used to.

SCREENING INSTRUMENTS: DEPRESSION (CONTINUED)

BECK DEPRESSION INVENTORY, SHORT FORM (CONTINUED)

K. Work difficulty
3 I can't do any work at all.
2 I have to push myself very hard to do anything.
1 It takes extra effort to get started at doing something.
0 I can work about as well as before.

L. Fatigability
3 I get too tired to do anything.
2 I get tired from doing anything.
1 I get tired more easily than I used to.
0 I don't get any more tired than usual.

M. Anorexia
3 I have no appetite at all anymore.
2 My appetite is much worse now.
1 My appetite is not as good as it used to be.
0 My appetite is no worse than usual.

Source: Reproduced with permission from Beck AT, Beck RW. Screening depressed patients in family practice: A rapid technic. Postgrad Med 1972;52:81.

GERIATRIC DEPRESSION SCALE

Choose the best answer for how you felt over the past week

1. Are you basically satisfied with your life?	yes / no
2. Have you dropped many of your activities and interests?	yes / no
3. Do you feel that your life is empty?	yes / no
4. Do you often get bored?	yes / no
5. Are you hopeful about the future?	yes / no
6. Are you bothered by thoughts you can't get out of your head?	yes / no
7. Are you in good spirits most of the time?	yes / no
8. Are you afraid that something bad is going to happen to you?	yes / no
9. Do you feel happy most of the time?	yes / no
10. Do you often feel helpless?	yes / no
11. Do you often get restless and fidgety?	yes / no
12. Do you prefer to stay at home, rather than going out and doing new things?	yes / no
13. Do you frequently worry about the future?	yes / no
14. Do you feel you have more problems with memory than most?	yes / no
15. Do you think it is wonderful to be alive now?	yes / no
16. Do you often feel downhearted and blue?	yes / no
17. Do you feel pretty worthless the way you are now?	yes / no
18. Do you worry a lot about the past?	yes / no
19. Do you find life very exciting?	yes / no
20. Is it hard for you to get started on new projects?	yes / no
21. Do you feel full of energy?	yes / no
22. Do you feel that your situation is hopeless?	yes / no
23. Do you think that most people are better off than you are?	yes / no

SCREENING INSTRUMENTS: DEPRESSION (CONTINUED)

GERIATRIC DEPRESSION SCALE (CONTINUED)

Choose the best answer for how you felt over the past week

24. Do you frequently get upset over little things?	yes / no
25. Do you frequently feel like crying?	yes / no
26. Do you have trouble concentrating?	yes / no
27. Do you enjoy getting up in the morning?	yes / no
28. Do you prefer to avoid social gatherings?	yes / no
29. Is it easy for you to make decisions?	yes / no
30. Is your mind as clear as it used to be?	yes / no

One point for each response suggestive of depression. (Specifically "no" responses to questions 1, 5, 7, 9, 15, 19, 21, 27, 29, and 30, and "yes" responses to the remaining questions are suggestive of depression.)

A score of ≥ 15 yields a sensitivity of 80% and a specificity of 100%, as a screening test for geriatric depression. Clin Gerontologist 1982;1:37.

Source: Reproduced with permission from Yesavage JA et al. Development and validation of a geriatric depression screening scale: A preliminary report. J Psychiatr Res 1982–83;17:37.

FUNCTIONAL ASSESSMENT SCREENING IN THE ELDERLY			
Target Area	**Assessment Procedure**	**Abnormal Result**	**Suggested Intervention**
Vision	Ask: "Do you have difficulty driving or watching television or reading or doing any of your daily activities because of your eyesight?" Test each eye with Jaeger card while patient wears corrective lenses (if applicable).	"Yes" and inability to read greater than 20/40	Refer to ophthalmologist.
Hearing	Whisper a short, easily answered question such as "What is your name?" in each ear while the examiner's face is out of direct view. Use audioscope set at 40 dB; test using 1,000 and 2,000 Hz.	Inability to answer question Inability to hear 1,000 or 2,000 Hz in both ears or inability to hear frequencies in either ear	Examine auditory canals for cerumen and clean if necessary. Repeat test; if still abnormal in either ear, refer for audiometry and possible prosthesis.
Arm	Proximal: "Touch the back of your head with both hands." Distal: "Pick up the spoon."	Inability to do task	Examine the arm fully (muscle, joint, and nerve), paying attention to pain, weakness, limited range of motion. Consider referral for physical therapy.
Leg	Observe the patient after instructing as follows: "Rise from your chair, walk 10 feet, return, and sit down."	Inability to complete task in 15 seconds	Do full neurologic and musculoskeletal evaluation, paying attention to strength, pain, range of motion, balance, and gait. Consider referral for physical therapy.
Continence of urine	Ask, "Do you ever lose your urine and get wet?" If yes, then ask, "Have you lost urine on at least 6 separate days?"	"Yes" to both questions	Ascertain frequency and amount. Search for remediable causes, including local irritations, polyuric states, and medications. Consider urologic referral.

	FUNCTIONAL ASSESSMENT SCREENING IN THE ELDERLY (CONTINUED)		
Target Area	**Assessment Procedure**	**Abnormal Result**	**Suggested Intervention**
Nutrition	Ask, "Without trying, have you lost 10 lb or more in the last 6 months?" Weigh the patient. Measure height.	"Yes" or weight is below acceptable range for height	Do appropriate medical evaluation.
Mental status	Instruct as follows: "I am going to name three objects (pencil, truck, book). I will ask you to repeat their names now and then again a few minutes from now."	Inability to recall all three objects after 1 minute	Administer Folstein Mini Mental State Examination. If score is less than 24, search for causes of cognitive impairment. Ascertain onset, duration, and fluctuation of overt symptoms. Review medications. Assess consciousness and affect. Do appropriate laboratory tests.
Depression	Ask, "Do you often feel sad or depressed?" or "How are your spirits?"	"Yes" or "Not very good, I guess"	Administer Geriatric Depression Scale. If positive (score above 15), check for antihypertensive, psychotropic, or other pertinent medications. Consider appropriate pharmacologic or psychiatric treatment.
ADL-IADL[a]	Ask, "Can you get out of bed yourself?" "Can you dress yourself?" "Can you make your own meals?" "Can you do your own shopping?"	"No" to any question	Corroborate responses with patient's appearance; question family members if accuracy is uncertain. Determine reasons for the inability (motivation compared with physical limitation). Institute appropriate medical, social, or environmental interventions.

FUNCTIONAL ASSESSMENT SCREENING IN THE ELDERLY (CONTINUED)

Target Area	Assessment Procedure	Abnormal Result	Suggested Intervention
Home environment	Ask, "Do you have trouble with stairs inside or outside of your home?" Ask about potential hazards inside the home with bathtubs, rugs, or lighting.	"Yes"	Evaluate home safety and institute appropriate countermeasures.
Social support	Ask, "Who would be able to help you in case of illness or emergency?"	—	List identified persons in the medical record. Become familiar with available resources for the elderly in the community.

[a]Activities of Daily Living–Instrumental Activities of Daily Living.

Source: Modified from Lachs MS et al. A simple procedure for screening for functional disability in elderly patients. Ann Intern Med 1990;112:699.

Geriatrics at your fingertips online edition 2007–2008. (http://www.geriatricsatyourfingertips.org, accessed 7/18/07)

95TH PERCENTILE OF BLOOD PRESSURE FOR BOYS

Age (y)	SBP (mm Hg) by percentile of height							DBP (mm Hg) by percentile of height						
	5%	10%	25%	50%	75%	90%	95%	5%	10%	25%	50%	75%	90%	95%
3	104	105	107	109	110	112	113	63	63	64	65	66	67	67
4	106	107	109	111	112	114	115	66	67	68	69	70	71	71
5	108	109	110	112	114	115	116	69	70	71	72	73	74	74
6	109	110	112	114	115	117	117	72	72	73	74	75	76	76
7	110	111	113	115	117	118	119	74	74	75	76	77	78	78
8	111	112	114	116	118	119	120	75	76	77	78	79	79	80
9	113	114	116	118	119	121	121	76	77	78	79	80	81	81
10	115	116	117	119	121	122	123	77	78	79	80	81	81	82
11	117	118	119	121	123	124	125	78	78	79	80	81	82	82
12	119	120	122	123	125	127	127	78	79	80	81	82	82	83
13	121	122	124	126	128	129	130	79	79	80	81	82	83	83
14	124	125	127	128	130	132	132	80	80	81	82	83	84	84
15	126	127	129	131	133	134	135	81	81	82	83	84	85	85
16	129	130	132	134	135	137	137	82	83	83	84	85	86	87
17	131	132	134	136	138	139	140	84	85	86	87	87	88	89

95TH PERCENTILE OF BLOOD PRESSURE FOR GIRLS

Age (y)	SBP (mm Hg) by percentile of height							DBP (mm Hg) by percentile of height						
	5%	10%	25%	50%	75%	90%	95%	5%	10%	25%	50%	75%	90%	95%
3	104	104	105	107	108	109	110	65	66	66	67	68	68	69
4	105	106	107	108	110	111	112	68	68	69	70	71	71	72
5	107	107	108	110	111	112	113	70	71	71	72	73	73	74
6	108	109	110	111	113	114	115	72	72	73	74	74	75	76
7	110	111	112	113	115	116	116	73	74	74	75	76	76	77
8	112	112	114	115	116	118	118	75	75	75	76	77	78	78
9	114	114	115	117	118	119	120	76	76	76	77	78	79	79
10	116	116	117	119	120	121	122	77	77	77	78	79	80	80
11	118	118	119	121	122	123	124	78	78	78	79	80	81	81
12	119	120	121	123	124	125	126	79	79	79	80	81	82	82
13	121	122	123	124	126	127	128	80	80	80	81	82	83	83
14	123	123	125	126	127	129	129	81	81	81	82	83	84	84
15	124	125	126	127	129	130	131	82	82	82	83	84	85	85
16	125	126	127	128	130	131	132	82	82	83	84	85	85	86
17	125	126	127	129	130	131	132	82	83	83	84	85	85	86

Source: http://www.nhlbi.nih.gov/guidelines/hypertension/child_tbl.htm (accessed 7/18/07).

BODY MASS INDEX CONVERSION TABLE		
Height in inches (cm)	**BMI 25 kg/m²**	**BMI 27 kg/m²**	**BMI 30 kg/m²**
	Body weight in pounds (kg)		
58 (147.32)	119 (53.98)	129 (58.51)	143 (64.86)
59 (149.86)	124 (56.25)	133 (60.33)	148 (67.13)
60 (152.40)	128 (58.06)	138 (62.60)	153 (69.40)
61 (154.94)	132 (59.87)	143 (64.86)	158 (71.67)
62 (157.48)	136 (61.69)	147 (66.68)	164 (74.39)
63 (160.02)	141 (63.96)	152 (68.95)	169 (76.66)
64 (162.56)	145 (65.77)	157 (71.22)	174 (78.93)
65 (165.10)	150 (68.04)	162 (73.48)	180 (81.65)
66 (167.64)	155 (70.31)	167 (75.75)	186 (84.37)
67 (170.18)	159 (72.12)	172 (78.02)	191 (86.64)
68 (172.72)	164 (74.39)	177 (80.29)	197 (89.36)
69 (175.26)	169 (76.66)	182 (82.56)	203 (92.08)
70 (177.80)	174 (78.93)	188 (85.28)	207 (93.90)
71 (180.34)	179 (81.19)	193 (87.54)	215 (97.52)
72 (182.88)	184 (83.46)	199 (90.27)	221 (100.25)
73 (185.42)	189 (85.73)	204 (92.53)	227 (102.97)
74 (187.96)	194 (88.00)	210 (95.26)	233 (105.69)
75 (190.50)	200 (90.72)	216 (97.98)	240 (108.86)
76 (193.04)	205 (92.99)	221 (100.25)	246 (111.59)

Metric conversion formula = weight (kg)/height (m²)

Example of BMI calculation:
A person who weighs 78.93 kilograms and is 177 centimeters tall has a BMI of 25: weight (78.93 kg)/height (1.77 m²) = 25

Non-metric conversion formula = [weight (pounds)/height (inches²)] × 704.5

Example of BMI calculation:
A person who weighs 164 pounds and is 68 inches (or 5' 8") tall has a BMI of 25: [weight (164 pounds)/height (68 inches²)] × 704.5 = 25

Source: Adapted from NHLBI Obesity Guidelines in Adults. (http://www.nhlbi.nih.gov/guidelines/obesity/bmi_tbl.htm) BMI on-line calculator: http://www.nhlbisupport.com/bmi.

ESTIMATE OF 10-YEAR CARDIAC RISK FOR MEN[a]

Age (y)	Points
20–34	–9
35–39	–4
40–44	0
45–49	3
50–54	6
55–59	8
60–64	10
65–69	11
70–74	12
75–79	13

Total Cholesterol	Points				
	Age 20–39	Age 40–49	Age 50–59	Age 60–69	Age 70–79
<160	0	0	0	0	0
160–199	4	3	2	1	0
200–239	7	5	3	1	0
240–279	9	6	4	2	1
≥ 280	11	8	5	3	1

	Points				
	Age 20–39	Age 40–49	Age 50–59	Age 60–69	Age 70–79
Nonsmoker	0	0	0	0	0
Smoker	8	5	3	1	1

HDL (mg/dL)	Points
≥ 60	–1
50–59	0
40–49	1
< 40	2

Systolic BP (mm Hg)	If Untreated	If Treated
< 120	0	0
120–129	0	1
130–139	1	2
140–159	1	2
≥ 160	2	3

Point Total	10-Year Risk %	Point Total	10-Year Risk %
< 0	< 1	9	5
0	1	10	6
1	1	11	8
2	1	12	10
3	1	13	12
4	1	14	16
5	2	15	20
6	2	16	25
7	3	≥ 17	≥ 30
8	4		10-Year Risk ____ %

[a]Framingham point scores.
Source: U.S. Department of Health and Human Services, Public Health Service, National Institutes of Health, National Heart, Lung, and Blood Institute. NIH Publication No. 01-3305, May 2001.
On-line risk calculator: http://hp2010.nhlbihin.net/atpiii/calculator.asp?usertype=prof.

ESTIMATE OF 10-YEAR CARDIAC RISK FOR WOMEN[a]

Age (y)	Points				
20–34	–7				
35–39	–3				
40–44	0				
45–49	3				
50–54	6				
55–59	8				
60–64	10				
65–69	12				
70–74	14				
75–79	16				

Total Cholesterol	Points				
	Age 20–39	Age 40–49	Age 50–59	Age 60–69	Age 70–79
<160	0	0	0	0	0
160–199	4	3	2	1	1
200–239	8	6	4	2	1
240–279	11	8	5	3	2
≥ 280	13	10	7	4	2

	Points				
	Age 20–39	Age 40–49	Age 50–59	Age 60–69	Age 70–79
Nonsmoker	0	0	0	0	0
Smoker	9	7	4	2	1

HDL (mg/dL)	Points
≥ 60	–1
50–59	0
40–49	1
< 40	2

Systolic BP (mm Hg)	If Untreated	If Treated
< 120	0	0
120–129	1	3
130–139	2	4
140–159	3	5
≥ 160	4	6

Point Total	10-Year Risk %	Point Total	10-Year Risk %
< 9	< 1	17	5
9	1	18	6
10	1	19	8
11	1	20	11
12	1	21	14
13	2	22	17
14	2	23	22
15	3	24	27
16	4	≥ 25	≥ 30

10-Year Risk _____%

[a]Framingham point scores.
Source: U.S. Department of Health and Human Services, Public Health Service, National Institutes of Health, National Heart, Lung, and Blood Institute. NIH Publication No. 01-3305, May 2001.
On-line risk calculator: http://hp2010.nhlbihin.net/atpiii/calculator.asp?usertype=prof.

ESTIMATE OF 10-YEAR STROKE RISK FOR MEN

Age (y)	Points	Untreated Systolic Blood Pressure (mm Hg)	Points
54–56	0	97–105	0
57–59	1	106–115	1
60–62	2	116–125	2
63–65	3	126–135	3
66–68	4	136–145	4
69–72	5	146–155	5
73–75	6	156–165	6
76–78	7	166–175	7
79–81	8	176–185	8
82–84	9	186–195	9
85	10	196–205	10

Treated Systolic Blood Pressure (mm Hg)	Points	History of Diabetes	Points
97–105	0	No	0
106–112	1	Yes	2
113–117	2		
118–123	3		
124–129	4		
130–135	5		
136–142	6		
143–150	7		
151–161	8		
162–176	9		
177–205	10		

Cigarette Smoking	Points	Cardiovascular Disease	Points
No	0	No	0
Yes	3	Yes	4

Atrial Fibrillation	Points	Left Ventricular Hypertrophy on Electrocardiogram	Points
No	0	No	0
Yes	4	Yes	5

Point Total	10-Year Risk %	Point Total	10-Year Risk %
1	3	16	22
2	3	17	26
3	4	18	29
4	4	19	33
5	5	20	37
6	5	21	42
7	6	22	47
8	7	23	52
9	8	24	57
10	10	25	63
11	11	26	68
12	13	27	74
13	15	28	79
14	17	29	84
15	20	30	88

10-Year Risk _____%

Source: Modified Framingham Stroke Risk Profile. Circulation 2006;113:e873–923.

ESTIMATE OF 10-YEAR STROKE RISK FOR WOMEN

Age (y)	Points	Untreated Systolic Blood Pressure (mm Hg)	Points
54–56	0	95–106	1
57–59	1	107–118	2
60–62	2	119–130	3
63–64	3	131–143	4
65–67	4	144–155	5
68–70	5	156–167	6
71–73	6	168–180	7
74–76	7	181–192	8
77–78	8	193–204	9
79–81	9	205–216	10
82–84	10		

Treated Systolic Blood Pressure (mm Hg)	Points	History of Diabetes	Points
95–106	1	No	0
107–113	2	Yes	3
114–119	3		
120–125	4		
126–131	5		
132–139	6		
140–148	7		
149–160	8		
161–204	9		
205–216	10		

Cigarette Smoking	Points	Cardiovascular Disease	Points
No	0	No	0
Yes	3	Yes	2

Atrial Fibrillation	Points	Left Ventricular Hypertrophy on Electrocardiogram	Points
No	0	No	0
Yes	6	Yes	4

Point Total	10-Year Risk %	Point Total	10-Year Risk %
1	1	16	19
2	1	17	23
3	2	18	27
4	2	19	32
5	2	20	37
6	3	21	43
7	4	22	50
8	4	23	57
9	5	24	64
10	6	25	71
11	8	26	78
12	9	27	84
13	11	28	
14	13	29	10-Year Risk _____ %
15	16	30	

Source: Modified Framingham Stroke Risk Profile. Circulation 2006;113:e873–923.

Recommended Immunization Schedule for Persons Aged 0–6 Years—UNITED STATES · 2007

Vaccine ▼ / Age ►	Birth	1 month	2 months	4 months	6 months	12 months	15 months	18 months	19–23 months	2–3 years	4–6 years
Hepatitis B[1]	HepB	HepB			HepB						
Rotavirus[2]			Rota	Rota	Rota						
Diphtheria, Tetanus, Pertussis[3]			DTaP	DTaP	DTaP		DTaP				DTaP
Haemophilus influenzae type b[4]			Hib	Hib	Hib[4]	Hib					
Pneumococcal[5]			PCV	PCV	PCV	PCV				PCV · PPV	
Inactivated Poliovirus			IPV	IPV	IPV		IPV				IPV
Influenza[6]					Influenza (Yearly)						
Measles, Mumps, Rubella[7]						MMR					MMR
Varicella[8]						Varicella					Varicella
Hepatitis A[9]						HepA (2 doses)				HepA Series	
Meningococcal[10]										MPSV4	

Legend:
- Range of recommended ages
- Catch-up immunization
- Certain high-risk groups

see footnote 1

HepB Series

This schedule indicates the recommended ages for routine administration of currently licensed childhood vaccines, as of December 1, 2006, for children aged 0–6 years. Additional information is available at http://www.cdc.gov/nip/recs/child-schedule.htm. Any dose not administered at the recommended age should be administered at any subsequent visit, when indicated and feasible. Additional vaccines may be licensed and recommended during the year. Licensed combination vaccines may be used whenever any components of the combination are indicated and other components of the vaccine are not contraindicated and if approved by the Food and Drug Administration for that dose of the series. Providers should consult the respective Advisory Committee on Immunization Practices statement for detailed recommendations. Clinically significant adverse events that follow immunization should be reported to the Vaccine Adverse Event Reporting System (VAERS). Guidance about how to obtain and complete a VAERS form is available at http://www.vaers.hhs.gov or by telephone, 800-822-7967. FOOTNOTES ON REVERSE SIDE

DEPARTMENT OF HEALTH AND HUMAN SERVICES
CENTERS FOR DISEASE CONTROL AND PREVENTION
SAFER · HEALTHIER · PEOPLE™

The Recommended Immunization Schedules for Persons Aged 0–18 Years are approved by:
Advisory Committee on Immunization Practices (http://www.cdc.gov/nip/acip)
American Academy of Pediatrics (http://www.aap.org)
American Academy of Family Physicians (http://www.aafp.org)

More information regarding vaccines, administration can be obtained from the websites above or the CDC-INFO contact center:

800-CDC-INFO
ENGLISH & ESPAÑOL – 24/7
[800-232-4636]

Keep track of your child's immunizations with the CDC Childhood Immunization Scheduler
www.cdc.gov/nip/kidstuff/scheduler.htm

FOOTNOTES

1. Hepatitis B vaccine (HepB). (*Minimum age: birth*)

At birth:

- Administer monovalent HepB to all newborns before hospital discharge.
- If mother is hepatitis surface antigen (HBsAg)-positive, administer HepB and 0.5 mL of hepatitis B immune globulin (HBIG) within 12 hours of birth.
- If mother's HBsAg status is unknown, administer HepB within 12 hours of birth. Determine the HBsAg status as soon as possible and if HBsAg-positive, administer HBIG (no later than age 1 week).
- If mother is HBsAg-negative, the birth dose can only be delayed with physician's order and mother's negative HBsAg laboratory report documented in the infant's medical record.

After the birth dose:

- The HepB series should be completed with either monovalent HepB or a combination vaccine containing HepB. The second dose should be administered at age 1–2 months. The final dose should be administered at age ≥ 24 weeks. Infants born to HBsAg-positive mothers should be tested for HBsAg and antibody to HBsAg after completion of ≥ 3 doses of a licensed HepB series, at age 9–18 months (generally at the next well-child visit).

4-month dose:

- It is permissible to administer 4 doses of HepB when combination vaccines are administered after the birth dose. If monovalent HepB is used for doses after the birth dose, a dose at age 4 months is not needed.

2. Rotavirus vaccine (Rota). (*Minimum age: 6 weeks*)

- Administer the first dose at age 6–12 weeks. Do not start the series later than age 12 weeks.
- Administer the final dose in the series by age 32 weeks. Do not administer a dose later than age 32 weeks.
- Data on safety and efficacy outside of these age ranges are insufficient.

3. Diphtheria and tetanus toxoids and acellular pertussis vaccine (DTaP). (*Minimum age: 6 weeks*)

- The fourth dose of DTaP may be administered as early as age 12 months, provided 6 months have elapsed since the third dose.
- Administer the final dose in the series at age 4–6 years.

4. *Haemophilus influenzae* type b conjugate vaccine (Hib). (*Minimum age: 6 weeks*)

- If PRP-OMP (PedvaxHIB® or ComVax® [Merck]) is administered at ages 2 and 4 months, a dose at age 6 months is not required.
- TriHiBit® (DTaP/Hib) combination products should not be used for primary immunization but can be used as boosters following any Hib vaccine in children aged ≥ 12 months.

5. Pneumococcal vaccine. (*Minimum age: 6 weeks for pneumococcal conjugate vaccine [PCV]; 2 years for pneumococcal polysaccharide vaccine [PPV]*)

- Administer PCV at ages 24–59 months in certain high-risk groups. Administer PPV to children aged ≥ 2 years in certain high-risk groups. See MMWR 2000;49(No. RR-9):1–35.

6. Influenza vaccine. (*Minimum age: 6 months for trivalent inactivated influenza vaccine [TIV]; 5 years for live, attenuated influenza vaccine [LAIV]*)

- All children aged 6–59 months and close contacts of all children aged 0–59 months are recommended to receive influenza vaccine.
- Influenza vaccine is recommended annually for children aged ≥ 59 months with certain risk factors, health-care workers, and other persons (including household members) in close contact with persons in groups at high risk. See MMWR 2006;55(No. RR-10):1–41.
- For healthy persons aged 5–49 years, LAIV may be used as an alternative to TIV.
- Children receiving TIV should receive 0.25 mL if aged 6–35 months or 0.5 mL if aged ≥ 3 years.
- Children aged < 9 years who are receiving influenza vaccine for the first time should receive 2 doses (separated by ≥ 4 weeks for TIV and ≥ 6 weeks for LAIV).

7. Measles, mumps, and rubella vaccine (MMR). (*Minimum age: 12 months*)

- Administer the second dose of MMR at age 4–6 years. MMR may be administered before age 4–6 years, provided ≥ 4 weeks have elapsed since the first dose and both doses are administered at age ≥ 12 months.

8. Varicella vaccine. (*Minimum age: 12 months*)

- Administer the second dose of varicella vaccine at age 4–6 years. Varicella vaccine may be administered before age 4–6 years, provided that ≥ 3 months have elapsed since the first dose and both doses are administered at age ≥ 12 months. If second dose was administered ≥ 28 days following the first dose, the second dose does not need to be repeated.

9. Hepatitis A vaccine (HepA). (*Minimum age: 12 months*)

- HepA is recommended for all children aged 1 year (ie, aged 12–23 months). The 2 doses in the series should be administered at least 6 months apart.
- Children not fully vaccinated by age 2 years can be vaccinated at subsequent visits.
- HepA is recommended for certain other groups of children, including in areas where vaccination programs target older children. See MMWR 2006;55(No. RR-7):1–23.

10. Meningococcal polysaccharide vaccine (MPSV4). (*Minimum age: 2 years*)

- Administer MPSV4 to children aged 2–10 years with terminal complement deficiencies or anatomic or functional asplenia and certain other high-risk groups. See MMWR 2005;54 (No. RR-7):1–21.

Recommended Immunization Schedule for Persons Aged 7–18 Years—UNITED STATES • 2007

Vaccine ▼ Age ►	7–10 years	11–12 YEARS	13–14 years	15 years	16–18 years
Tetanus, Diphtheria, Pertussis[1]	see footnote 1	Tdap		Tdap	
Human Papillomavirus[2]	see footnote 2	HPV (3 doses)		HPV Series	
Meningococcal[3]	MPSV4	MCV4		MCV4[3] MCV4	
Pneumococcal[4]		PPV			
Influenza[5]		Influenza (Yearly)			
Hepatitis A[6]		HepA Series			
Hepatitis B[7]		HepB Series			
Inactivated Poliovirus[8]		IPV Series			
Measles, Mumps, Rubella[9]		MMR Series			
Varicella[10]		Varicella Series			

Legend:
- Range of recommended ages
- Catch-up immunization
- Certain high-risk groups

This schedule indicates the recommended ages for routine administration of currently licensed childhood vaccines, as of December 1, 2006, for children aged 7–18 years. Additional information is available at http://www.cdc.gov/nip/recs/child-schedule.htm. Any dose not administered at the recommended age should be administered at any subsequent visit, when indicated and feasible. Additional vaccines may be licensed and recommended during the year. Licensed combination vaccines may be used whenever any components of the combination are indicated and other components of the vaccine are not contraindicated and if approved by the Food and Drug Administration for that dose of the series. Providers should consult the respective Advisory Committee on Immunization Practices statement for detailed recommendations. Clinically significant adverse events that follow immunization should be reported to the Vaccine Adverse Event Reporting System (VAERS). Guidance about how to obtain and complete a VAERS form is available at http://www.vaers.hhs.gov or by telephone, 800-822-7967. FOOTNOTES ON REVERSE SIDE

DEPARTMENT OF HEALTH AND HUMAN SERVICES
CENTERS FOR DISEASE CONTROL AND PREVENTION
SAFER·HEALTHIER·PEOPLE™

The Recommended Immunization Schedules for Persons Aged 0–18 Years are approved by:

Advisory Committee on Immunization Practices (http://www.cdc.gov/nip/acip)
American Academy of Pediatrics (http://www.aap.org)
American Academy of Family Physicians (http://www.aafp.org)

More information regarding vaccines administered can be obtained from the websites above or the CDC-INFO contact center:

800-CDC-INFO
ENGLISH & ESPAÑOL · 24/7

[800-232-4636]

Keep track of your child's immunizations with the
CDC Childhood Immunization Scheduler
www.cdc.gov/nip/kidstuff/scheduler.htm

FOOTNOTES

1. Tetanus and diphtheria toxoids and acellular pertussis vaccine (Tdap). (*Minimum age: 10 years for BOOSTRIX® and 11 years for ADACEL™*)

- Administer at age 11–12 years for those who have completed the recommended childhood DTP/DTaP vaccination series and have not received a tetanus and diphtheria toxoids vaccine (Td) booster dose.
- Adolescents aged 13–18 years who missed the 11–12 year Td/Tdap booster dose should also receive a single dose of Tdap if they have completed the recommended childhood DTP/DTaP vaccination series.

2. Human papillomavirus vaccine (HPV). (*Minimum age: 9 years*)

- Administer the first dose of the HPV vaccine series to females at age 11–12 years.
- Administer the second dose 2 months after the first dose and the third dose 6 months after the first dose.
- Administer the HPV vaccine series to females at age 13–18 years if not previously vaccinated.

3. Meningococcal vaccine. (*Minimum age: 11 years for meningococcal conjugate vaccine [MCV4]; 2 years for meningococcal polysaccharide vaccine [MPSV4]*)

- Administer MCV4 at age 11–12 years and to previously unvaccinated adolescents at high school entry (at approximately age 15 years).
- Administer MCV4 to previously unvaccinated college freshmen living in dormitories; MPSV4 is an acceptable alternative.
- Vaccination against invasive meningococcal disease is recommended for children and adolescents aged ≥ 2 years with terminal complement deficiencies or anatomic or functional asplenia and certain other high-risk groups. See MMWR 2005;54(No. RR-7):1–21. Use MPSV4 for children aged 2–10 years and MCV4 or MPSV4 for older children.

4. Pneumococcal polysaccharide vaccine (PPV). (*Minimum age: 2 years*)

- Administer for certain high-risk groups. See MMWR 1997;46(No. RR-8):1–24, and MMWR 2000;49(No. RR-9):1–35.

5. Influenza vaccine. (*Minimum age: 6 months for trivalent inactivated influenza vaccine [TIV]; 5 years for live, attenuated influenza vaccine [LAIV]*)

- Influenza vaccine is recommended annually for persons with certain risk factors, health-care workers, and other persons (including household members) in close contact with persons in groups at high risk. See MMWR 2006;55 (No. RR-10):1–41.
- For healthy persons aged 5–49 years, LAIV may be used as an alternative to TIV.
- Children aged < 9 years who are receiving influenza vaccine for the first time should receive 2 doses (separated by ≥ 4 weeks for TIV and ≥ 6 weeks for LAIV).

6. Hepatitis A vaccine (HepA). (*Minimum age: 12 months*)

- The 2 doses in the series should be administered at least 6 months apart.
- HepA is recommended for certain other groups of children, including in areas where vaccination programs target older children. See MMWR 2006;55 (No. RR-7):1–23.

7. Hepatitis B vaccine (HepB). (*Minimum age: birth*)

- Administer the 3-dose series to those who were not previously vaccinated.
- A 2-dose series of Recombivax HB® is licensed for children aged 11–15 years.

8. Inactivated poliovirus vaccine (IPV). (*Minimum age: 6 weeks*)

- For children who received an all-IPV or all-oral poliovirus (OPV) series, a fourth dose is not necessary if the third dose was administered at age ≥ 4 years.
- If both OPV and IPV were administered as part of a series, a total of 4 doses should be administered, regardless of the child's current age.

9. Measles, mumps, and rubella vaccine (MMR). (*Minimum age: 12 months*)

- If not previously vaccinated, administer 2 doses of MMR during any visit, with ≥ 4 weeks between the doses.

10. Varicella vaccine. (*Minimum age: 12 months*)

- Administer 2 doses of varicella vaccine to persons without evidence of immunity.
- Administer 2 doses of varicella vaccine to persons aged < 13 years at least 3 months apart. Do not repeat the second dose, if administered ≥ 28 days after the first dose.
- Administer 2 doses of varicella vaccine to persons aged ≥ 13 years at least 4 weeks apart.

Recommended Adult Immunization Schedule, by Vaccine and Age Group
UNITED STATES • OCTOBER 2007–SEPTEMBER 2008

Vaccine	Age group (yrs)		
	19–49	50–64	≥65
Tetanus, diphtheria, pertussis (Td/Tdap)[1]*	1-dose Td booster every 10 yrs		
	Substitute 1 dose of Tdap for Td		
Human papillomavirus (HPV)[2]*	3 doses (females) (0, 2, 6 mos)		
Measles, mumps, rubella (MMR)[3]*	1 or 2 doses	1 dose	
Varicella[4]*	2 doses (0, 4–8 wks)		
Influenza[5]*	1 dose annually	1 dose annually	
Pneumococcal (polysaccharide)[6,7]	1–2 doses		1 dose
Hepatitis A[8]*	2 doses (0, 6–12 mos, or 0, 6–18 mos)		
Hepatitis B[9]*	3 doses (0, 1–2, 4–6 mos)		
Meningococcal[10]*	1 or more doses		
Zoster[11]			1 dose

*Covered by the Vaccine Injury Compensation Program.

NOTE: This schedule must be read along with the footnotes, which can be found at www.cdc.gov/nip/recs/adult-schedule.htm

For all persons in this category who meet the age requirements and who lack evidence of immunity (e.g., lack documentation of vaccination or have no evidence of prior infection)	Recommended if some other risk factor is present (e.g., on the basis of medical, occupational, lifestyle, or other indications)

This schedule indicates the recommended age groups and medical indications for routine administration of currently licensed vaccines for persons aged ≥19 years, as of October 1, 2007. Licensed combination vaccines may be used whenever any components of the combination are indicated and when the vaccine's other components are not contraindicated. For detailed recommendations on all vaccines, including those used primarily for travelers or that are issued during the year, consult the manufacturers' package inserts and the complete statements from the Advisory Committee on Immunization Practices (www.cdc.gov/nip/publications/acip-list.htm).

Report all clinically significant postvaccination reactions to the Vaccine Adverse Event Reporting System (VAERS). Reporting forms and instructions on filing a VAERS report are available at www.vaers.hhs.gov or by telephone, 800-822-7967.

Information on how to file a Vaccine Injury Compensation Program claim is available at www.hrsa.gov/vaccinecompensation or by telephone, 800-338-2382. To file a claim for vaccine injury, contact the U.S. Court of Federal Claims, 717 Madison Place, N.W., Washington, D.C. 20005; telephone, 202-357-6400.

Additional information about the vaccines in this schedule and contraindications for vaccination is also available at www.cdc.gov or from the CDC-INFO Contact Center at 800-CDC-INFO (800-232-4636) in English and Spanish, 24 hours a day, 7 days a week.

Recommended Adult Immunization Schedule, by Vaccine and Medical and Other Indications
UNITED STATES • OCTOBER 2007–SEPTEMBER 2008

Vaccine	Pregnancy	Immuno-compromising conditions (excluding human immunodeficiency virus [HIV]), medications[13], radiation[13]	HIV infection[3,12,13] CD4+ T lymphocyte count <200 cells/μL	HIV infection[3,12,13] CD4+ T lymphocyte count ≥200 cells/μL	Diabetes, heart disease, chronic pulmonary disease, chronic alcoholism	Asplenia[12] (including elective splenectomy and terminal complement component deficiencies)	Chronic liver disease	Kidney failure, end-stage renal disease, receipt of hemodialysis	Health-care personnel
Tetanus, diphtheria, pertussis (Td/Tdap)[1]*	1 dose Td booster every 10 yrs								
			Substitute 1 dose of Tdap for Td						
Human papillomavirus (HPV)[2]*		3 doses for females through age 26 yrs (0, 2, 6 mos)							
Measles, mumps, rubella (MMR)[3]*	Contraindicated	Contraindicated	Contraindicated			1 or 2 doses			
Varicella[4]*	Contraindicated	Contraindicated	Contraindicated			2 doses (0, 4–8 wks)			
Influenza[5]*	1 dose TIV annually								1 dose TIV or LAIV annually
Pneumococcal (polysaccharide)[6,7]						1–2 doses			
Hepatitis A[8]*							2 doses (0, 6–12 mos, or 0, 6–18 mos)		
Hepatitis B[9]*							3 doses (0, 1–2, 4–6 mos)		
Meningococcal[10]*						1 or more doses			
Zoster[11]	Contraindicated	Contraindicated	Contraindicated		1 dose				

For all persons in this category who meet the age requirements and who lack documentation of vaccination or have no evidence of prior infection

Recommended if some other risk factor is present (e.g., on the basis of medical, occupational, lifestyle, or other indications)

* Covered by the Vaccine Injury Compensation Program.

NOTE: This schedule must be read along with the footnotes, which can be found at www.cdc.gov/nip/recs/adult-schedule.htm

Approved by
the Advisory Committee on Immunization Practices,
the American College of Obstetricians and Gynecologists,
the American Academy of Family Physicians,
and the American College of Physicians

DEPARTMENT OF HEALTH AND HUMAN SERVICES
CENTER FOR DISEASE CONTROL AND PREVENTION

PROFESSIONAL SOCIETIES & GOVERNMENTAL AGENCIES

Abbreviation	Full Name	Internet Address
AACE	American Association of Clinical Endocrinologists	http://www.aace.com
AAD	American Academy of Dermatology	http://www.aad.org
AAFP	American Academy of Family Physicians	http://www.aafp.org
AAHPM	American Academy of Hospice and Palliative Medicine	http://www.aahpm.org
AAN	American Academy of Neurology	http://www.aan.com/professionals
AAO	American Academy of Ophthalmology	http://www.aao.org
AAO-HNS	American Academy of Otolaryngology–Head and Neck Surgery	http://www.entnet.org
AAOS	American Academy of Orthopaedic Surgeons	http://www.aaos.org
AAP	American Academy of Pediatrics	http://www.aap.org
ACC	American College of Cardiology	http://www.acc.org
ACCP	American College of Chest Physicians	http://www.chestnet.org
ACG	American College of Gastroenterology	http://www.acg.gi.org
ACIP	Advisory Committee on Immunization Practices	http://www.cdc.gov/vaccines/recs/acip
ACOG	American College of Obstetricians and Gynecologists	http://www.acog.com
ACP	American College of Physicians	http://www.acponline.org
ACPM	American College of Preventive Medicine	http://www.acpm.org
ACR	American College of Radiology	http://www.acr.org
ACR	American College of Rheumatology	http://www.rheumatology.org
ACS	American Cancer Society	http://www.cancer.org
ACSM	American College of Sports Medicine	http://www.acsm.org
ADA	American Diabetes Association	http://www.diabetes.org
AGA	American Gastroenterological Association	http://www.gastro.org

PROFESSIONAL SOCIETIES & GOVERNMENTAL AGENCIES (CONTINUED)

Abbreviation	Full Name	Internet Address
AGS	American Geriatrics Society	http://www.americangeriatrics.org
AHA	American Heart Association	http://www.americanheart.org
AHRQ	Agency for Healthcare Research and Quality	http://www.ahrq.gov
AMA	American Medical Association	http://www.ama-assn.org
ANA	American Nurses Association	http://www.nursingworld.org
AOA	American Optometric Association	http://www.aoa.org
ASA	American Stroke Association	http://www.strokeassociation.org
ASAM	American Society of Addiction Medicine	http://www.asam.org
ASCCP	American Society for Colposcopy and Cervical Pathology	http://www.asccp.org
ASCO	American Society of Clinical Oncology	http://www.asco.org
ASCRS	American Society of Colon and Rectal Surgeons	http://www.fascrs.org
ASGE	American Society for Gastrointestinal Endoscopy	http://asge.org
ASHA	American Speech-Language-Hearing Association	http://www.asha.org
ASN	American Society of Neuroimaging	http://www.asnweb.org
ATA	American Thyroid Association	http://www.thyroid.org
ATS	American Thoracic Society	http://www.thoracic.org
AUA	American Urological Association	http://auanet.org
BASHH	British Association for Sexual Health and HIV	http://www.bashh.org
	Bright Futures	http://brightfutures.org
BSAC	British Society for Antimicrobial Chemotherapy	http://www.bsac.org.uk
CDC	Centers for Disease Control and Prevention	http://www.cdc.gov
COG	Children's Oncology Group	http://www.childrensoncologygroup.org

PROFESSIONAL SOCIETIES & GOVERNMENTAL AGENCIES (CONTINUED)		
Abbreviation	**Full Name**	**Internet Address**
CSVS	Canadian Society for Vascular Surgery	http://csvs.vascularweb.org
CTF	Canadian Task Force on Preventive Health Care	http://www.ctfphc.org
EASD	European Association for the Study of Diabetes	http://www.easd.org
ERS	European Respiratory Society	http://ersnet.org
ESC	European Society of Cardiology	http://www.escardio.org
ESCDPCP	European and Other Societies on Cardiovascular Disease Prevention in Clinical Practice	http://www.escardio.org
ESH	European Society of Hypertension	http://www.eshonline.org
IARC	International Agency for Research on Cancer	http://screening.iarc.fr
ICSI	Institute for Clinical Systems Improvement	http://www.icsi.org
IDF	International Diabetes Federation	http://www.idf.org
NAPNAP	National Association of Pediatric Nurse Practitioners	http://www.napnap.org
NCI	National Cancer Institute	http://www.cancer.gov/cancerinformation
NEI	National Eye Institute	http://www.nei.nih.gov
NGC	National Guideline Clearinghouse	http://www.guidelines.gov
NHLBI	National Heart, Lung, and Blood Institute	http://www.nhlbi.nih.gov
NHPCO	National Hospice and Palliative Care Organization	http://www.nhpco.org
NIAAA	National Institute on Alcohol Abuse and Alcoholism	http://www.niaaa.nih.gov
NICE	National Institute for Health and Clinical Excellence	http://www.nice.org.uk
NIDCR	National Institute of Dental and Craniofacial Research	http://www.nidr.nih.gov
NIHCDC	National Institutes of Health Consensus Development Conference	http://www.consensus.nih.gov

PROFESSIONAL SOCIETIES & GOVERNMENTAL AGENCIES (CONTINUED)		
Abbreviation	**Full Name**	**Internet Address**
NIP	National Immunization Program	http://www.cdc.gov/nip
NOF	National Osteoporosis Foundation	http://www.nof.org
NTSB	National Transportation Safety Board	http://www.ntsb.gov
SCF	Skin Cancer Foundation	http://www.skincancer.org
SGIM	Society for General Internal Medicine	http://www.sgim.org
SVU	Society for Vascular Ultrasound	http://www.svunet.org
UK-NHS	United Kingdom National Health Service	http://www.nhs.uk
USPSTF	United States Preventive Services Task Force	http://www.ahrq.gov/clinic/uspstfix.htm
WHO	World Health Organization	http://www.who.int/en

Index